Essential Clinical Pharmacology

Essential Clinical Pharmacology

Peter Lewis
MA, MD, PhD, MRCP

Senior Lecturer in Clinical Pharmacology
Royal Postgraduate Medical School
University of London

Honorary Consultant Physician to
Hammersmith Hospital London
and
Queen Charlotte's Hospital London

MTP PRESS LIMITED · LANCASTER · ENGLAND
International Medical Publishers

Published by
MTP Press Limited
Falcon House
Lancaster, England

First published 1981

British Library Cataloguing in Publication Data
Lewis, Peter
Essential clinical pharmacology.
1. Pharmacology
I. Title
615'.7 RM300
ISBN 978-0-85200-372-5 ISBN 978-94-011-7243-1 (eBook)
DOI 10.1007/978-94-011-7243-1

Phototypesetting by Swiftpages Ltd., Liverpool

Contents

Preface vii

Section 1: Introduction to Therapeutics

1 Essentials of clinical pharmacology 3
2 Names and classes of drugs 14
3 Adverse effects of drugs 17

Section 2: Chemotherapy

4 Drugs and infectious disease 25
5 Tuberculosis and tropical diseases 34
6 Drugs and the immune system 38
7 Cancer chemotherapy 44

Section 3: The Central Nervous System

8 Drugs and the central nervous system 51
9 Anaesthetics 54
10 Analgesics 60
11 Hypnotics 65
12 Antiepileptics 68
13 Psychotropic drugs 72
14 Parkinson's disease 77
15 Social and addictive drugs 81

Section 4: The Autonomic Nervous System
16 Drugs and the autonomic nervous system 87
17 Antihypertensives 95
18 Cardiac drugs 102
19 Drugs for asthma 108

Section 5: Hormones and Pregnancy
20 The endocrine system 113
21 Diabetes mellitus 119
22 Oral contraception 124
23 Drugs and pregnancy 128

Section 6: The Kidney and the Gut
24 Diuretics and the kidney 135
25 Drugs and the digestive system 139

Section 7: The Blood
26 Drugs and anaemia 147
27 Anticoagulation 150

Section 8: Topical Therapy
28 Drugs and the skin 157
29 Drugs and the eye 161

Section 9: Ward Therapeutics
30 Drugs and emergencies 165
31 Drugs and regulations 170

Index 175

Preface

This book is about drugs and how they are used in the treatment of disease. The development of effective drugs is one of the wonders of our century. It is difficult to believe that so few of the medicines we now use routinely were available when our grandparents were children. The last 50 years has seen an astonishing burst of discoveries – antibiotics, antihypertensives, antiarrhythmics, psychotropics, anticonvulsants, steroids and many others.

Of course this pace of advance has brought problems. Modern drugs are more powerful than the remedies they replaced, so it takes more skill and knowledge to use them correctly. Therapeutics has had to become more disciplined and now relies heavily on clinical pharmacology, which is the science of drugs in man.

The tradition of this series of books has been to answer the questions an intelligent person would ask about a particular subject. Conventional texts on pharmacology can seem rather dull catalogues of drugs. Of course it is important to identify a drug, but it seems of greater importance to know how drugs work, how they are chosen for particular patients, what problems they produce and why. In this book the Socratic question and answer format has been deliberately chosen to bring out this sort of information.

Peter Lewis

SECTION 1

INTRODUCTION TO THERAPEUTICS

1

Essentials of clinical pharmacology

What is clinical pharmacology?

Pharmacology is the study of drugs, and clinical pharmacology is the study of drugs in man. Although drugs have been used for the treatment of illnesses since time immemorial, clinical pharmacology has only recently been established as a separate scientific discipline. The purpose of clinical pharmacology is to bridge the gap between the laboratory pharmacologist who develops drugs, and the clinicians who use them. The stimulus to develop clinical pharmacology came in the 1950s when the explosion of new drug discoveries created the need for detailed clinical evaluation of drugs and the knowledge necessary to regulate drug usage.

What is a drug?

A drug can be widely defined as any chemical capable of affecting living processes, or narrowly defined as a substance recognized in an official formulary for the diagnosis, prophylaxis or treatment of disease.

How do drugs work?

In the past, drugs were thought to exert a magical influence on the body and the ingredients of medicines were chosen more for their mystical associations than for their therapeutic effects. No rational physical explanation for the action of a drug was expected nor sought. Even today vestiges of this superstitious attitude towards drugs remain. New cancer cures are enthusiastically greeted by the public, and native herbal remedies still exert a fascination out of proportion to their clinically known effects. It is widely appreciated that at least a part of many drug effects may be exerted not by pharmacology but by the power of suggestion. Inert tablets, if administered with conviction, often have quite profound effects on patients. This is known as the placebo effect.

However, genuine reproducible drug effects depend on biochemical

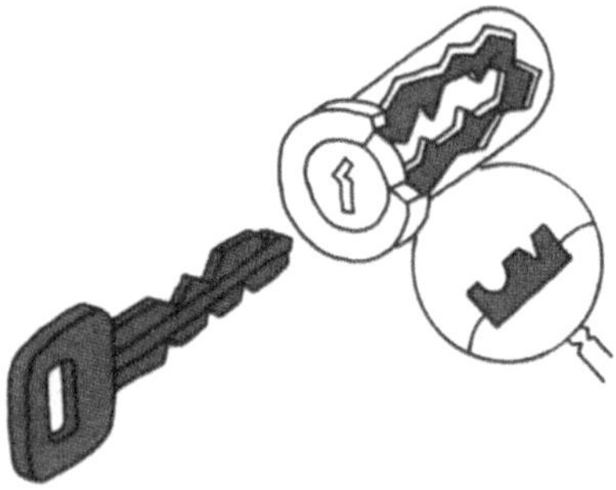

A convenient analogy is that of a car and its ignition key:

The engine of the car is started when the ignition key is inserted into the ignition lock and turned.

Likewise, many cellular processes only start when specific 'keys' combine with 'locks' in cells. Cells contain many such 'locks' (receptors), each sensitive to its own particular 'key'. Normally, the 'keys' are compounds such as hormones and neurotransmitters.

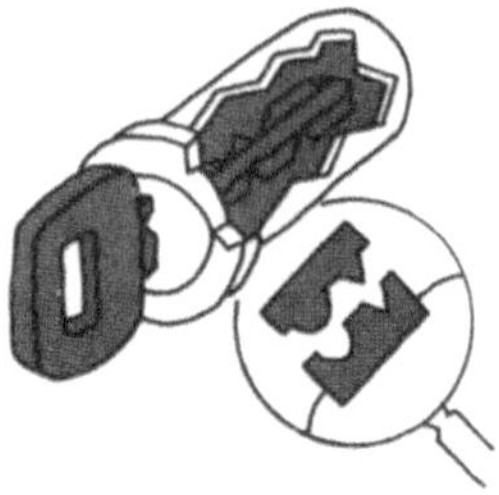

The ignition key is designed specifically to fit the car lock. Its particular cross-sectional pattern allows it to fit the lock, while the pattern on the face allows the key to turn and so start the engine.

Cellular receptors, too, are specific by virtue of their shape.

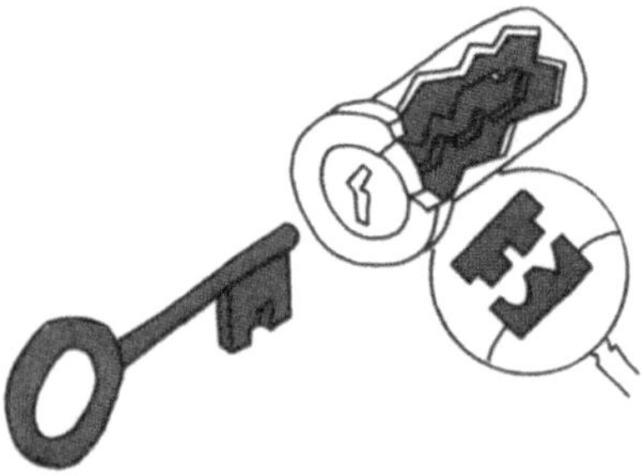

Other sorts of key normally will not fit the car lock.

Similarly, most cellular receptors only accept one hormone.

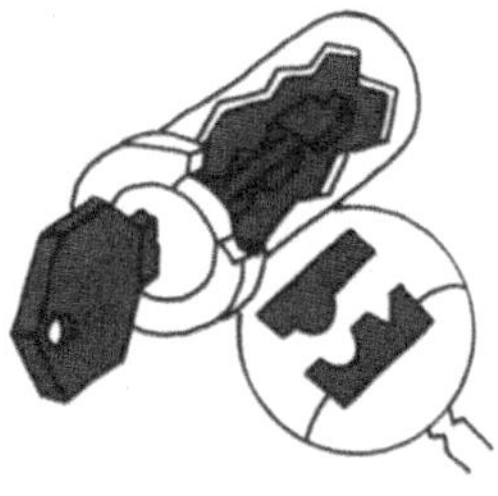

Sometimes keys of a similar, but not identical, structure also start the car.

In the same way, closely related compounds can activate receptors, so that it is possible to design chemicals that 'fit' a receptor such that they work just as well as the naturally occurring 'key'.

Figure 1 Drug-receptor interaction. Courtesy of Dr Rod Flower

events within the body. Drugs act on living cells by virtue of their chemical activity. In order to exert these effects the drugs need to be transported to their site of action within the body, an aspect of drug action which has been increasingly studied in recent years.

How do drugs affect cells?

There are believed to be two sorts of interaction between drugs and cells, specific and non-specific. In the first the drug combines with a specific receptor substance (Figure 1). By attaching itself to this receptor, the drug takes the place of a natural molecule and hence interrupts the cell's normal activities. Originally all drug receptors were thought to be sited on the outside of cells, i.e. on the cell membrane, their usual receptor function being to test their environment for neurotransmitters or hormones; these are the chemical messengers which are released by other body cells as part of the body's complex communication system. Recently it has become apparent that similar drug effects can occur with receptor molecules within cells. Enzymes or other large molecules inside cells can be the site of drug attachment. In such specific interactions, the structure of the drug is critical, and even small changes in the chemical configuration of a drug molecule can considerably alter its effects.

In a non-specific drug interaction, the drug does not combine with a specific receptor molecule but alters cellular function in a more crude and general way. In drugs having this sort of action chemical structural changes are less important. For example, general anaesthetics are fat soluble substances which may depress nerve cell function simply by dissolving in the nerve cell membrane and disrupting its usual excitability. The study of how drugs act is called *pharmacodynamics*.

How do drugs get to their site of action?

Drugs move around the body using the body's own transport processes. Drugs are usually small molecules which dissolve in the watery matrix of tissues, diffusing from areas of high concentration to areas of low concentration. Drug molecules often become attached or bound to body proteins, especially within the blood and this leads to differences in the concentration of available drug in different tissues. Like the natural constituents of the body, drugs are rapidly distributed around the organs of the body via the circulatory system. The absorption and distribution of a drug and the way in which the drug is eliminated from the body are processes which have a profound effect on drug action. Obviously if the drug is having a chemical effect on cells then the concentration of drug at the site of action is critical. How quickly the drug reaches its target and how rapidly it is removed determines the dose and frequency of administration which is needed to produce the desired effect. The science which deals with drug movement in the body is called *pharmacokinetics*. Pharmacokinetics deals with three vital processes: drug absorption, drug distribution and drug elimination from the body.

How are drugs absorbed and distributed?

Drug administration essentially consists of placing a high concentration of drug at some site in or on the body. From the site of administration, the drug diffuses into the adjacent tissue, dissolves in tissue fluid, drains into the vascular system and is then carried around the body by the blood. Once within the blood the drug is available for diffusion into any body region. In some organs the drug is actually transported out of the blood by carrier systems; this happens particularly in the liver and the kidney. Some organs are relatively impervious to the entry of a drug. For example, the blood vessels in the brain do not allow the entry of certain drugs, the cells lining the cerebral blood vessels constituting a physical blood–brain barrier.

Obviously a qualitative description of drug absorption and distribution is no use in predicting what would happen with particular drugs. Measurement of concentrations of drug in various body fluids at different times after administration enables the pharmacokinetics of the drug to be studied, and in this way predictions can be made about the rapidity with which therapeutic concentrations of drugs are obtained in different organs.

How are drugs eliminated from the body?

Two processes are usually involved in drug elimination: metabolism and excretion. In the simplest case, i.e. excretion, the drug is not chemically metabolized in the body but is simply directed into some body fluid and eliminated. This can occur if the drug is excreted by the kidney in the urine or taken up by the liver and secreted into the bile. Usually, however, the process of elimination is speeded up because the drug is metabolized, that is, changed into another substance by an active chemical process. Usually the process of metabolism makes the drug more easily eliminated by the kidney or the liver. Some drugs have many different metabolites. Occasionally the metabolites of the drug can have a more profound effect on the body than the original drug; this is known as drug activation. However, the process of metabolism is usually that of detoxification and the metabolites are less active, less fat soluble and less able to diffuse around the body.

How do these considerations influence drug dosages?

How much of a drug is given to a patient and how frequently is usually fairly standard for most drugs. However, when a new drug is first introduced dose and dosage intervals have to be determined by measuring plasma concentrations of the drug after various doses (Figure 2a) and measuring the rate of elimination of the drug from the blood

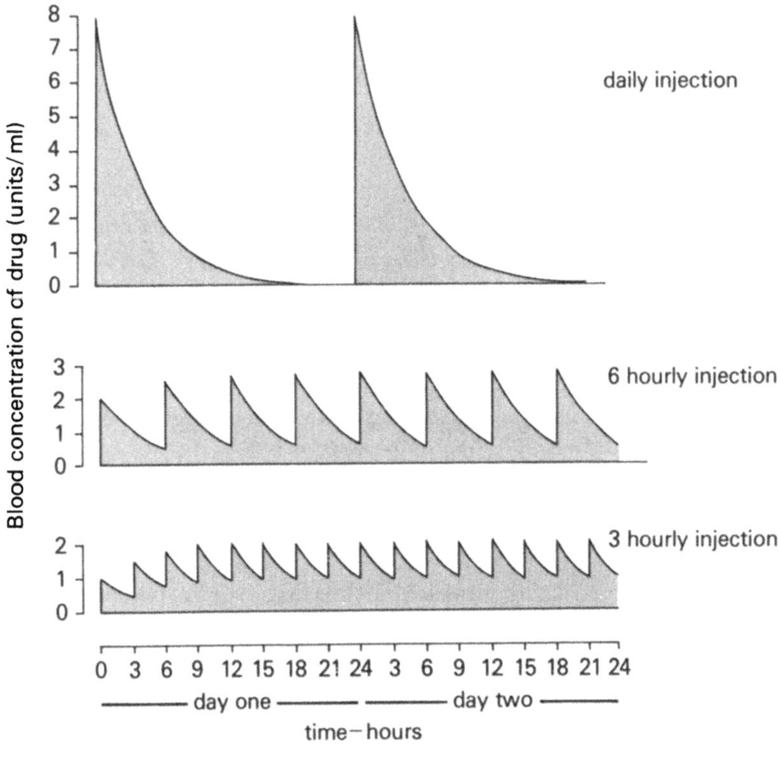

(a)

Figure 2(a) Effect of dosage interval on blood levels of a drug. The drug is an antibiotic with a short halflife, 3 hours. It is given intravenously. The figure shows the blood levels which would be produced if the same dose of drug were given as one injection, or split up and given every 6 hours or every 3 hours. If it were necessary for treatment to have a blood level of 1 unit/ml only the 3 hourly regime would be effective, and if the drug were toxic in concentrations of 5 units/ml the daily injection would be dangerous

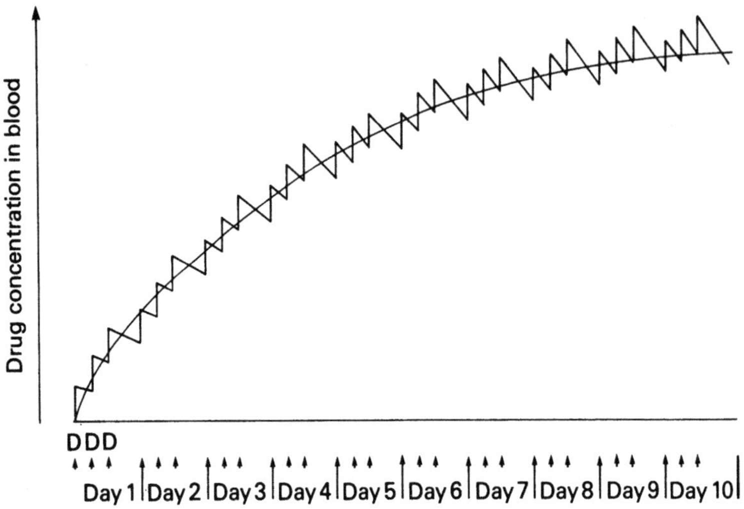

(b)

Figure 2(b) Cumulation of a drug. If a drug has a long elimination halflife and is administered frequently then cumulation occurs. The figure shows the accumulation of drug which would occur if a drug with a halflife of 48 hours were given 3 times a day (↑). A plateau concentration is eventually reached, but it takes 10 days and the amount of drug accumulated is much greater than when the treatment is initiated

(Figure 2b). It is usual to measure the time taken for the plasma concentration of the drug to fall by one half of its initial value after a single dose; this time is called the *halflife*. Some drugs have a short halflife of minutes or even seconds while for other drugs excretion is slow and the halflife is prolonged, hours or even days. The frequency at which drugs are dosed depends on their halflife. Drugs rapidly eliminated from the blood with a short halflife need to be administered frequently or continuously in order to maintain adequate concentrations in the blood and target tissues. On the other hand, drugs which are slowly eliminated need to be given at infrequent intervals if they are not to accumulate. Too frequent administration results in high concentrations of the drug building up, which might lead to toxicity.

Do all patients require the same dose?

Unfortunately there is a great deal of variation between individuals in their response to drugs, even when the doses are adjusted to take into account differences in body weight. Most of these differences are not mysterious idiosyncrasies but can be explained by differences in the rates at which drugs are eliminated in different individuals. A lot of these differences in elimination rates are hereditary or genetic. Hence identical twins tend to eliminate drugs at the same rate, because they have identical enzyme systems in their livers and identical kidney function. The most marked differences in drug handling occur in disease. Some drugs like digoxin are entirely eliminated by excretion in the urine. If the patient has renal impairment then the rate of elimination of digoxin is grossly altered. Similar considerations apply to patients with liver disease who are often unable to metabolize drugs effectively. Such considerations have to be taken into account when doses are calculated for patients with hepatic or renal disease.

Do some drugs have to be individually tailored to patients?

Very much so. We have mentioned the problem of renal and hepatic disease. However, in some cases where the actual concentration of drug is critical, dosage has to be tailored to achieve exactly the right therapeutic concentration. For example, in the treatment of epilepsy it is known that fits are best suppressed with fewest side-effects if the drug concentrations in blood are kept within certain precise limits, the so-called therapeutic range. In order to achieve this, measurements of drug concentration have to be made in individual patients, and then their dose of drug adjusted up or down to get them into the right range. There are many examples of drug doses which need to be very carefully adjusted. These include digoxin and gentamicin. Fortunately, however, for the majority of drugs there is a wide range of concentration in body tissues which is both effective and not too toxic. It is this flexibility which allows us to use standard doses at standard dosage intervals in patients of different body size with probably very different drug elimination rates. Some of the main factors which produce variation between patients are listed in Table 1.

Table 1 Some differences between patients which affect their responses to drugs

Compliance	– Some patients take the drugs as prescribed, many do not.
Absorption	– Can vary in completeness and rate even from an injection site.
Metabolism	– Genetic differences in metabolic routes and rates, effect of other drugs on liver metabolism, liver disease, age of patient.
Elimination	– Differences in renal function.
Psychological	– Some patients show a striking placebo response to treatment. Neurotic patients get more imagined side-effects.

How are drugs administered?

Almost every conceivable route has been used to administer drugs to the patient. The alimentary tract is the most popular and drugs can be administered under the tongue, swallowed or administered as a suppository into the rectum. The lungs can be used to administer drugs which are presented as gases, vapours or aerosols. Drugs can be injected into the body either subcutaneously, intramuscularly, intravenously, into the cerebrospinal fluid or the epidural space. Drugs can also be given topically, that is to say directly to the affected organ which usually means the skin but can mean into the eyes, ears or nose, into the vagina or injected into joints, bladder or peritoneal cavity. It should not be forgotten that the object of drug administration is to get the drug safely to the target site where its actions will have a therapeutic effect.

How can one drug influence the action of another?

Drug interactions are frequent and most patients with a significant medical condition end up taking several different drugs. Indeed the

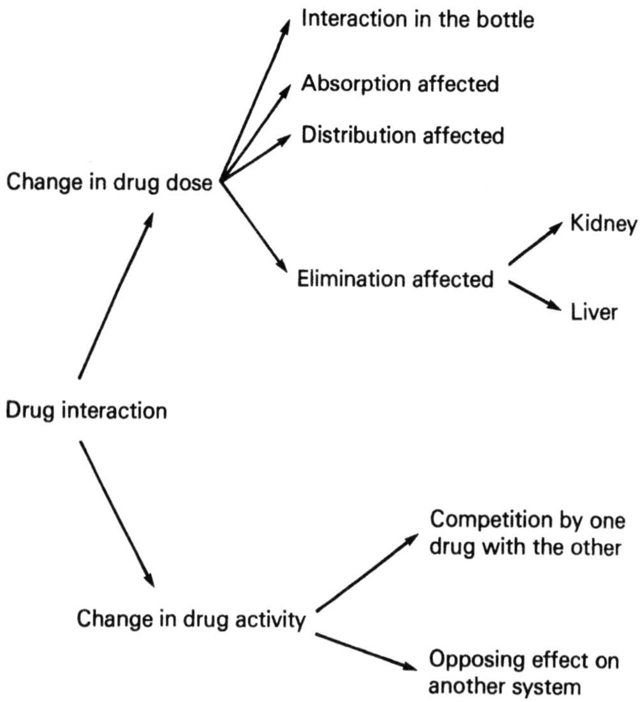

Figure 3 How drugs may interact

average number of drugs taken by a patient in hospital is five. Such multiple drug usage leads to complications and the frequency of adverse reactions to drugs increases with the number of drugs taken. Interactions with important drugs can also be caused when the patient takes some trivial 'over-the-counter' remedy, which he believes to be harmless because it is readily available at the chemist.

There are many different sorts of interaction (Figure 3). Drugs can be incompatible if mixed together in an injection, one drug may retard absorption of another, drugs can alter the rate at which the liver metabolizes and one drug can directly antagonize another. Some of these processes are obvious and indeed we use them as part of our everyday experience, for example using coffee to overcome the drowsiness induced by alcohol. In rare cases drug interactions can be very severe or even fatal. Such interactions usually involve drugs where the dose is critical, such as anticoagulants or antihypertensives.

Why are there so many different ways of administering drugs?

Many considerations affect the routes chosen to administer a drug. The most important of these are:

(1) Convenience. If at all possible drugs should be given orally. An injection carries with it the risk of infection and some discomfort.

(2) Effectiveness. Some drugs are just not absorbed when given by mouth, and must be administered by injection or inhalation. For example, heparin and insulin are broken down by digestive enzymes in the stomach, and hence have to be given by subcutaneous or intramuscular injection. Obviously gases can only be absorbed via the lung.

(3) Selectivity. Certain routes of administration allow a high concentration of drug to be obtained at the site of action without exposing the rest of the body to a high concentration. In some cases any other means of administration would be totally impractical. Examples of this would be giving local anaesthetics directly around a sensory nerve, using eye drops to obtain a high local concentration of mydriatic in the eye and using some drugs sublingually. When drugs are given sublingually rather than swallowed, they are absorbed directly into the blood stream without having to go through the portal system into the liver. As the liver is the main metabolizing organ in the body, this means that less of the drug is broken down when given sublingually.

(4) Speed of action. Drugs have much quicker systemic action when they are given intravenously than when they are taken orally,

because there is no delay in absorption into the blood. Drugs given intramuscularly or by inhalation are also rapidly effective.

(5) Safety. Any injection carries the risk of some infection being carried into the tissues and, by virtue of the speed of onset of effect, an injection is more dangerous. Every route has its particular hazards. For example, it is unwise to use antibiotics on the skin as this more commonly leads to allergy to the drug than when it is given orally.

What is the difference between a pill, a tablet and a capsule?

Modern medicines are carefully formulated so that they are consistent in their effects. The rate at which a pill or capsule releases its drug into the alimentary canal and allows it to be absorbed into the blood can vary depending on how the drug is formulated, what excipients it is mixed with and so on. Pills and tablets are solid formulations which must dissolve before absorption can occur.

Capsules contain powdered drug which is more rapidly absorbed once the capsule is dissolved in the gut. Spansules provide for a prolonged absorption time, as the different particles inside the capsule are coated with compounds of different dissolution times.

Slow release formulation tablets have been devised so that drugs can have a more prolonged effect after their administration. Slow absorption is usually achieved by incorporating the drug in a wax or plastic base from which it leaches out at a slow rate.

Should oral drugs be taken on an empty stomach?

If a drug is taken after a meal it is absorbed slowly, first because it may be bound to the food and held in the gut, and secondly because the drug passes more slowly from the stomach into the intestine. Drugs are more rapidly absorbed if they are given on an empty stomach and this is to be preferred, unless the drug is one which causes some gastro-intestinal upset in which case this can be minimized if the drug is taken with food. For most drugs this is not a critical matter but tetracycline is an example of a drug whose absorption is affected by food. It should not be taken with or after food, particularly milk, as this reduces its absorption.

How are drugs developed?

One hundred years ago practically all drugs were natural products extracted from plants; nowadays most drugs are synthetic chemicals.

New drugs are first tested on animals and on isolated animal organs in what is known as a screening process. Substances which show interesting pharmacological actions progress to further tests which determine their spectrum of action. Biochemical studies are also needed on interesting molecules to find out how the drug is absorbed and how it is metabolized and excreted. Before an interesting new drug can be tested in man, its toxicity is evaluated by prolonged animal testing. If the drug passes all these stages, and only a small proportion do, single doses of the drug can be given to human volunteers. These early clinical studies will show up any subjective side-effects and will indicate the dose in man which produces a measurable effect. Metabolism of the drug in man is usually slower than in animals and often different metabolites are formed in different species. If pilot trials in normal volunteers are promising, then the drug can be administered to patients suffering from the condition which it is hoped the drug will treat. The need here is to compare the new drug with a placebo to confirm that it really does have a therapeutic action. It is important to rule out bias on the patients' and the investigator's part by adoption of a 'double blind technique'. In such trials neither the patient nor the investigator know whether placebo or active drug is being administered, and the results of the trial are not known until the code is broken at the end of the study.

How do we know drugs are safe?

No drug is entirely without side-effects. In therapeutics one looks at the risk to benefit ratio in deciding whether the treatment is more likely to do good than harm. Licensing of drugs for use in medicine is regulated in most countries, and before a drug can be marketed evidence of efficacy and relative lack of toxicity has to be presented to the appropriate authorities. In recent years this process has become more and more bureaucratic, and there are now fears that excessive regulation of drug safety is diminishing the number of new drugs being produced by the pharmaceutical industry.

2

Names and classes of drugs

How are drugs named?

Every drug has several different names, and some have a very large number. This profusion of names is often a source of confusion and can indeed be dangerous. The various names have different origins and uses.

Chemical name

There are precise rules for naming chemical compounds, and the chemical name defines the structure of the drug molecule. Because of this the chemical name of a drug is complex and unsuitable for use in prescribing.

Approved name (or generic)

The approved name is the official name given to the drug. It is usually a short name based on the drug's chemical structure and has the advantage that related drugs have similar names. The approved name is the one which should be used in prescribing.

Proprietary or trade name

The proprietary name is the commercial name given to the drug by the pharmaceutical company which makes and promotes it. Newer drugs are only protected by patent for a few years after their introduction so it is important for the manufacturer to firmly establish the trade name during this period so that when it is out of patent the drug will continue earning revenue. After the patent period runs out, other manufacturers can market the drug and usually introduce new trade names, resulting in the same drug marketed under many different names. Table 2 shows some of the various names for some common drugs.

Table 2 Chemical, approved (generic) and proprietary names of some common drugs

Usual proprietary name	*Chemical name*	*Approved (generic) name*
Mogadon	2,3,Dihydro-7-nitro-5-phenyl-1 *H*-1,4-benzodiazepin-2-one	Nitrazepam
Panadol	*N*-Acetyl-*p*-aminophenol	Paracetamol
Lasix	4-Chloro-*N*-furfuryl-5 sulphamoylanthranilic acid	Frusemide
Fluothane	2-Bromo-2-chloro-1,1,1-trifluoroethane	Halothane
Inderal	(±)-1-Isopropylamino-3-naphth-1′-yloxypropan-2-ol hydrochloride	Propranolol

What names ought to be used in prescribing?

There are arguments both for and against the use of proprietary names. The advantage of using a proprietary name is that one ensures a standard product from one manufacturer will be supplied to the patient, and that there can be no substitute made for a cheaper brand of the drug which may not behave in exactly the same way. For example, different brands of drugs dissolve at different rates, and for certain drugs like digoxin where dosage is critical, this can be important. However some of the force of this argument is dissipated, because all drugs which are now marketed in the UK have to fulfil certain standard requirements of purity and formulation.

In general, the single approved name is to be preferred as it makes for a more sure identification of the drug, and because it is more informative and scientific. Additionally, the approved name is the one which is referred to in scientific literature and in pharmacology textbooks. Finally the drug marketed under an approved or generic name is usually less expensive than the same drug marketed under the proprietary name. Certainly in any examination situation the approved name of the drug should be used.

How can one find the approved name of a drug?

This may be difficult because manufacturers tend to flaunt their trade names and push the approved names into obscurity. However, it is mandatory in all drug advertisements for the approved name of the drug to appear, although it often appears in tiny characters. Various reference works contain lists which give the approved names of proprietary drugs. Perhaps the most widely used publication which lists all drugs in common use is MIMS, the Monthly Index of Medical Specialties. Although the drugs in MIMS are listed by proprietary name, there is an index which gives the approved name.

How are drugs classified?

A drug can be classified in many different ways depending on its origins, its chemical structure, its pharmacological action and its uses. In practice most traditional classifications of drugs are a hybrid of all these different systems which have grown up over the years. Thus antibiotics are classified by their chemical structure, e.g. penicillin and macrolide rather than by their particular drug usage, while oxytocic drugs are classified by their use rather than by their structures which are very different. β-Blockers and β-mimetics are classified by their pharmacological properties, activity of receptor action or other pharmacological actions. All of these classifications are a compromise. Therapeutics is a practical subject and drugs are studied primarily because they are useful, not out of purely academic interest. The different classifications we have tend to reflect the uses of drugs more than other considerations, and this is how it should be.

3

Adverse effects of drugs

What is an adverse drug effect?

The World Health Organization has defined an adverse effect of a drug as one which is noxious, unintended and occurs at doses normally used in man for prophylaxis, diagnosis or therapy.

How important are adverse effects of drugs?

The overall balance for drug treatment is strongly positive and much more good than harm comes from the use of modern drugs. However, some individual patients undoubtedly suffer badly from adverse effects, and it has been estimated that 5% of all hospital admissions are due to adverse effects of therapy. Furthermore, 1 in 200 of all deaths in hospital are thought to be caused by drug treatment rather than the disease being treated. These are worrying statistics since they measure obvious major events, and beneath the tip of this iceberg floats a mass of more trivial ill health caused by drugs. Prescribing physicians should constantly remember the first rule in therapeutics is *'primum non nocere'*, first do no harm; and that no drug has just one action.

In practice therapeutics is a matter of judging relative risks. Every drug administration carries some risk, the magnitude varying with the drug and the condition of the patient being treated. For serious conditions, a high risk of adverse effect is perfectly acceptable but for trivial conditions, only trivial risks can be tolerated. In all cases steps should be taken to minimize the risk of adverse reaction as described below.

What sorts of adverse effect are there?

Almost any medical condition can be caused by an adverse drug reaction, and this possibility must be kept in mind when patients develop new illnesses or symptoms during the course of drug treatment. The mechanisms of some adverse reactions are known so that a rational classification of adverse effects is possible. One classification of adverse effects is shown in Table 3. Some adverse reactions will occur in nearly all patients provided they are given the drug in a large enough amount for a long enough period. These reactions can be termed predictable and include exaggerated therapeutic effects, side-effects, toxic effects and cumulative overdosage. By contrast, other adverse effects are unpredictable, that is to say only a small proportion of patients will ever develop them no matter how much drug they receive. Some of these unpredictable effects are due to drug allergy and others to idiosyncrasy.

Table 3 Types of adverse effects

Predictable adverse effects	
(1)	Exaggerated therapeutic effect
(2)	Side-effects
(3)	Toxic effects
(4)	Cumulative toxicity
Unpredictable adverse effects	
(1)	Drug allergy
(2)	Idiosyncrasy

What is an exaggerated therapeutic effect?

Drugs are often employed to alter some physiological or biochemical variable in a patient, such as lowering blood pressure in hypertension, inhibiting blood coagulation in thrombosis, or lowering blood glucose levels in diabetes. Here the dose is critical; too little and the drug is ineffective, too much and an adverse effect results, e.g. faintness due to an excessive fall in blood pressure, bleeding due to overanticoagulation and coma due to hypoglycaemia. Unfortunately, judging the right dose is difficult due to differences between individuals and their response to a drug, due particularly to differences in the patient's handling of the drugs (see Chapter 1). Interactions between the different drugs the patient is taking can also lead to a relative overdose or underdose.

What are side-effects?

Side-effects are any effects produced by the drug other than the desired therapeutic response. They can be experienced by the patient as a symptom, e.g. nausea in a patient given morphine, or may occur without the patient being aware of them, as the onset of diabetes in a patient taking diuretics.

Side-effects occur because few drugs are specific and most produce many different effects in the body. The nearest thing to an ideal drug without side-effects are the hormones used as replacement therapy, e.g. L-thyroxine in myxoedema. Here the drug precisely corrects the defect in the patient and providing the dose of thyroxine is correctly adjusted, the treatment has no side-effects.

What is a toxic effect?

Most drugs are toxic or poisonous given in large enough doses. The ratio of the effective therapeutic dose and the dose where toxicity is noticed is called the *therapeutic ratio*. Drugs with a high therapeutic ratio are basically safe as they can be taken in relatively large doses without adverse effect. Examples would be ampicillin or the vitamins. Other drugs such as digoxin or warfarin have a low therapeutic ratio. Their dose is critical and merely by doubling the dose an adverse toxic effect can be produced.

What is cumulative toxicity?

Some drugs can cause adverse effects following prolonged dosing and toxicity is related to the total cumulative dose. For example, patients who have taken large doses of mild analgesics for many years may develop chronic renal failure. A large cumulative dose is necessary for this effect to occur. Cumulative toxicity also occurs after prolonged treatment with corticosteroids, chloroquine and phenothiazines. Cirrhosis of the liver in alcoholics is another example of the same phenomenon.

How does drug allergy occur?

Only a few patients exposed to a drug become allergic to it. Allergic reactions to a drug are not predictable, but atopic patients, who have eczema or asthma are more likely to develop them. It is thought that the basic mechanism in all cases is that the drug combines with a protein in the body to produce an antigen; and this antigen is capable of stimulating the immune system to produce an antibody against the drug. The type of drug allergy is thought to be related to the type of antibody that the body produces. Clinically, allergic reactions are very variable. Anaphylaxis is the worst type of allergic reaction and this can be fatal. Here the patient becomes shocked and collapses soon after challenge with the drug to which he has become allergic. Fortunately, drug allergy is usually much less dramatic, skin rashes being the commonest manifestation but haemolytic anaemia, liver diseases, renal failure and many other syndromes can be produced by an immune response to the drug. Once a patient has shown an allergic response to the drug, care must be taken to ensure that he does not receive it again because there is a risk of him developing an anaphylactic reaction should he be re-exposed. Therefore, it is important that drug allergy should be recorded in the case records, and that the patient should be told so he can mention it to any doctor treating him and wear or carry some notification. Allergies to antibiotics, sulphonamides, X-ray contrast media are the most common so it is well worth while to ask any patient about to receive an injection of these drugs if they are allergic to them, or, their companion if the patient is unconscious. Failure to take this simple precaution has cost lives in the past and will unfortunately continue to do so in the future.

What is a drug idiosyncrasy?

Idiosyncrasy is an unusual reaction to a drug, usually due to a genetic susceptibility. For example, some patients when exposed to a variety of drugs, including sulphonamides and aspirin, develop an acute haemolytic anaemia. These individuals can be shown to have red blood cells which are deficient in the enzyme G-6-PD. Here, the red cells are susceptible to haemolysis when exposed to certain drugs. The deficiency is inherited and is especially common in black people and in Europeans from the Mediterranean area. Individuals with a deficiency of pseudocholinesterase in their blood cannot metabolize suxamethonium, the muscle relaxant, so they experience prolonged paralysis after administration of this drug. This is another example of drug idiosyncrasy.

How are adverse effects of drugs detected?

Early in the life of the prospective drug, its toxicity is determined in laboratory animals. Drugs which are highly toxic in animals never reach the stage of human testing. For those drugs which show no toxicity in animals testing continues and at the stage of early human trials, particular attention is paid to side-effects and toxic effects. The problem really is the idiosyncratic side-effects, which by definition only occur in a small proportion of the population. The detection of these sort of adverse effects is only possible when the drug has been given to a large number of individuals. For this reason drugs are now often released for the first time onto the market on a basis 'monitored release'. Thus the first 5–10 000 patients who receive the drug are all followed up, and examined specifically to detect any unexpected problems. Despite these various precautions, drugs which have been used for years often turn out to have some unexpected side-effect, which someone has spotted by careful observation. The Committee on Safety of Medicines has a responsibility for monitoring the safety of drugs in the United Kingdom, and it encourages doctors who notice an adverse effect in their patients to report the incident on a special report form, the so-called yellow card system. The central collection of adverse drug reaction reports provides an important early warning system for adverse drug effects.

How can adverse drug reactions be minimized?

The first step is to educate prescribing doctors and the public, to ensure that drugs are only used when they are absolutely necessary. Secondly, once a drug is being used, the dose used should be the right one. In some cases of prolonged drug usage, the plasma concentration of the drug can be measured, and the dose adjusted to produce the optimum concentration of the drug in the plasma. For many drugs and those given for short periods of time, this is not practical, though there are certain rules of thumb which can be followed. The dose of drug should be smaller in children than in adults, and in old age drugs are handled less efficiently and a smaller dose is appropriate. Another important matter is whether the patient has any defect of liver or kidney function, which will allow the drug to accumulate in the body. For example, those drugs which are mainly metabolized in the liver, such as barbiturates and narcotics and steroids, need to be given in lower doses in patients with liver disease. Drugs which are mainly eliminated by the kidney, such as digoxin, should be given in lower doses to patients with renal failure. Finally, another important question is whether the patient is taking another drug with could interfere with the action of the second drug.

SECTION 2

CHEMOTHERAPY

4

Drugs and infectious disease

Why are some diseases infectious?

Only diseases caused by invasion of the body by living organisms are infectious. Infection consists of the transfer of the causative agent from an infected person to another susceptible individual. Some infections, such as smallpox, are extremely easily transferred between individuals; others such as leprosy, are of low infectivity and transfer of the disease only occurs after prolonged close contact between individuals. There are a number of diseases where it is still not known whether or not they are caused by infectious agents. A good example would be Hodgkin's lymphoma where family or community clustering of cases occurs, suggesting an infectious origin of the disease but no organism has as yet been positively identified.

What sort of organisms cause infectious disease?

There are a huge number of different infecting organisms, ranging from bacteria and viruses up to large complex animals such as nematode worms and insects. Infection with metozoa or multicelled animals is usually called infestation and the term infection reserved for diseases caused by micro-organisms. There are four main types of infective micro-organisms:

(1) Viruses and rickettsiae are elemental particles which take over the replicative mechanism of the host cells they colonize in order to reproduce. Viruses represent a particularly difficult problem for therapy as it is difficult to selectively kill the organism which so resembles the chromosomal elements of the living host cell. The only defences against viral infection are vaccination and quarantine. Rickettsiae are micro-organisms similar to viruses but rather larger. They are susceptible to attack with antibiotics, particularly tetracyclines.

(2) Bacteria are micro-organisms capable of independent existence, having a tough cell wall. They are conventionally classified according to whether they stain positively or negatively with Gram's stain and whether their usual form is oval, cocci or oblong, rods.

(3) Protozoa are unicellular organisms of a higher complexity than bacteria, in which the main constituents of a mammalian cell can be recognized. They are also capable of independent existence.

(4) Fungi are branching filamentous organisms also capable of an independent existence.

How is the causative agent for an infection identified?

It is only a hundred years or so (1881) since it was first convincingly demonstrated that human disease could be caused by a micro-organism. Robert Koch, a German pathologist, demonstrated that tuberculosis was due to the tubercle bacillus. Soon after this it was a brief hope that every human disease would be found to have a causative micro-organism which could be identified and eliminated. Unfortunately, micro-organisms are widely distributed so it was not always easy to determine whether the presence of a bacterium in a patient indicated that it was causing the disease or was merely an incidental bystander. Koch sorted out this situation by arguing that a true causative organism should be found in all cases of the disease and that after cultivation outside the body the organism could reproduce the disease when injected into a susceptible animal.

What measures are important in infectious disease?

The discovery of antibiotics, although extremely important, is not the main reason for the decrease in mortality from infectious disease this century. Public health measures based on prevention of infection have been far more important. These measures are designed to isolate individuals with infectious disease, to stop the spread of infection by disinfecting material from patients and to raise the immunity of the population against infectious diseases by immunization. Another measure to minimize infection is employing an aseptic technique in surgery, now universally adopted.

What drugs are useful in treating infections?

Drugs are used to combat infections in two ways, as supportive therapy and as chemotherapy. *Chemotherapy* is the use of drugs to directly attack the invading causative organism. *Supportive therapy* is aimed at controlling the manifestations of the disease, to improve the patient's condition and to allow time for the host's natural defences or for chemotherapy to control the infection. Typical supportive therapy would be antipyretic drugs to control fever, analgesic drugs to control pain, opiates to check diarrhoea and electrolyte solutions to replace lost fluid. In some infectious disorders we have no chemotherapy and supportive treatment is still most important.

What is chemotherapy?

Chemotherapy is the use of drugs which directly attack an infective agent without harm to the host. Ever since the first demonstration that some diseases were caused by infective bacteria pharmacologists have searched for drugs with such a selective action, toxic to the invader, harmless to man. Paul Ehrlich (1854–1915) called this concept 'the magic bullet' and synthesized the first such breakthrough substance, neoarsphenamine,* which was the first drug effective against syphilis.

Modern chemotherapy is now effective against more bacterial diseases but there are still few substances useful against viruses. Most chemotherapeutic agents are antibiotics which are, by definition, substances produced by living organisms, usually moulds, which are toxic to bacteria and other fungi. In many cases natural antibiotics have been chemically modified to give greater stability or selectivity of action. The substances so produced are called semi-synthetic antibiotics. Some chemotherapeutic substances, such as the sulphonamides or the nitrofurans are entirely synthetic and, strictly speaking, are not antibiotics.

How do chemotherapeutic drugs work?

The biochemistry of micro-organisms has many subtle differences from that of mammalian cells, and chemotherapy works by exploiting these differences. A classic example is the action of the sulphonamides. Sulphonamides are compounds similar in structure to *p*-aminobenzoic acid. Bacteria, but not mammalian cells, use *p*-aminobenzoic acid to form folic acid. Sulphonamides block the process and cause interruption of bacterial growth. Penicillins and cephalosporins both interfere with the formation of new cell walls in bacteria. Still other antibiotics, such as tetracyclines, chloramphenicol and streptomycin, interfere with bacterial ribosomes and so interrupt protein synthesis by the bacteria.

What are the different classes of antibiotics?

There are now many different antibiotics, and this is an active area of research with new agents frequently appearing. Antibiotics can be

* Neoarsphenamine is no longer used to treat syphilis, but it is still an ingredient in a brand of French toothpaste!

classified by their range of antimicrobial activity because different bacteria are attacked by different antibiotics. However, it is more usual to classify antibiotics according to their origin and chemical structure. There are five main groups and some subsidiary ones. The main groups are penicillins, cephalosporins, tetracyclines, aminoglycosides and sulphonamides. Other useful antibiotics which do not fit into this grouping are erythromycin, lincomycin, chloramphenicol and fusidic acid.

What is a broad-spectrum antibiotic?

Broad-spectrum antibiotics are effective against many different types of micro-organism and are useful in the clinical treatment of mixed infection. The tetracyclines and chloramphenicol have such a wide range of action, whereas most penicillins and aminoglycosides have a narrow antimicrobial spectrum.

How is an antibiotic selected for a patient?

The first decision is whether to treat with antibiotics. Antibiotics are not cure-alls and ideally they should only be given to patients with a proven infection, with an organism known to be sensitive to the proposed antibiotic. Unfortunately in the real world, this ideal situation is seldom seen. Probable bacterial infection is usually diagnosed on clinical grounds, and it may be difficult or impossible to isolate the infecting organism. In this situation an antibiotic is chosen which is likely to be effective against the usual organism causing the infection. For example, otitis media in children is usually caused by one of four different organisms. Since it is known that each of these bacteria is sensitive to amoxycillin this is the treatment usually chosen.

How are infective bacteria identified?

Occasionally bacteria can be identified directly by microscopic examination of specimens such as pus or centrifuged urine. Usually identification requires the organism to be grown in the laboratory. This is achieved by culturing specimens on the appropriate media. This can usually be done fairly rapidly, but there are practical difficulties. If the patient has been treated with any antibiotic prior to culture it is unusual to be able to identify the infective organism. The sensitivity to an antibiotic of a pathogenic bacterium in culture can be measured in various ways, the usual method being to place discs impregnated with different test antibiotics on the culture medium.

Why should antibiotics be used as little as possible?

When any drug is used risks and benefits have to be weighed up. Every antibiotic has some potential adverse effects on the patient. Unfortunately the more widely antibiotics are used, the more bacteria become resistant to them. It must be remembered that the body of the normal individual teems with colonizing bacteria on the skin, in the respiratory tract and in the alimentary canal. These bacteria can constitute the normal body flora. When an antibiotic is used it has a selective killing action, not only on the infecting organism but on the body flora as well. As sensitive bacteria in the normal flora are killed, other resistant organisms grow up to take their place. The normal balance of the body flora is altered. This imbalance can itself be harmful, and furthermore the resistant organisms can transfer their resistance to the antibiotic to other bacteria which are pathogenic or disease-producing.

How do bacteria become resistant to antibiotics?

Some bacteria are naturally resistant to certain antibiotics, for example, many bacteria produce an enzyme, penicillinase, which destroys penicillin and cephalosporin antibiotics. This type of resistance is innate and is present before the start of the treatment. However, another type of bacterial resistance may be acquired, i.e. it only arises because of the exposure to antibiotics. In a mixed population of bacteria exposed to an antibiotic, those few bacteria with resistance to the antibiotic are able to multiply rapidly. Capacity to resist the antibiotic is encoded on small packets of genetic material known as plasmids or R factors which can be transferred to other bacteria, even of quite different species. There are several different types of R factor, which confer different resistance patterns. Some enable bacteria to break down an antibiotic, others to prevent its uptake into the bacterial cell. Unfortunately some R factors confer resistance to several antibiotics at the same time. This capacity of a bacterial population to become resistant is most important, especially in hospitals where antibiotics are frequently used. Sometimes the only way to eliminate a dangerous resistant strain of bacteria is to avoid the use of certain antibiotics for a period of weeks or months. When the antibiotic is not used the bacteria with R factors gradually die out and the population becomes sensitive again.

What about prophylactic antibiotics?

In view of the resistance problem the need to keep antibiotic usage to a minimum is obvious. Using antibiotics to prevent an infection is not sensible as it leads to the early production of resistant organisms, and makes the potential infection more serious. Prophylactic antibiotics are therefore restricted to certain instances where they have been shown to confer a benefit. Patients who have congenital or rheumatic heart valve disease are at risk of contracting the serious infection bacterial endocarditis. The risk is highest when they are subjected to surgical procedures where bacteria escape into the blood stream; this occurs during dental treatment or childbirth. Patients with valvular heart disease are usually given antibiotic cover immediately before these events and for a short time afterwards, the object being to kill the bacteria before they can be established on the faulty heart valve. The only other common use of antibiotics as prophylaxis is in children who have had one attack of rheumatic fever. These children are usually put on prophylactic penicillin until they leave school to prevent a second infection with haemolytic streptococci.

What about antibiotics in the environment?

Unfortunately antibiotics are quite widely used in food production, both for veterinary treatment and as food additives allowing a more rapid growth of farm animals. Certain antibiotics improve the storage life of foods and are permitted as food additives. The use of antibiotics for all these purposes is regulated and a compromise has been worked out between the economies produced by antibiotics and the risk of promoting antibiotic resistant bacteria. Cows' milk is frequently contaminated with penicillin and in patients with penicillin allergy this can be important.

What side-effects are common to most antibiotics?

The most common problem with antibiotics is allergy. This can present as an acute emergency, particularly if the patient has been previously sensitized. The patient may develop cardiovascular failure and severe shortness of breath. Adrenaline, antihistamines and corticosteroids are used to treat such severe reactions. More commonly patients on antibiotics develop skin rashes. A patient who develops a skin rash from an antibiotic should not be given that antibiotic again as a more severe reaction may occur on a later occasion. Patients become allergic to antibiotics more readily if the antibiotic is directly applied to the skin, so antibiotic skin preparations are not a good idea.

The second most common side-effect of antibiotics is a gastro-intestinal disturbance with vomiting, nausea and, most common of all, diarrhoea. Many antibiotics irritate the mucosa of the gastro-intestinal tract. Some interfere with absorption from the gut and all of them upset the normal population of bacteria living in the intestine. Some degree of stomach upset is usual during any antibiotic treatment. This usually only amounts to some slight looseness of the bowels. On occasion, however, these reactions can be much more severe leading to a condition that resembles ulcerative colitis. Antibiotics can interfere with absorption of other drugs from the intestine. Women on the contraceptive pill sometimes develop breakthrough bleeding when given a course of antibiotics, and unwanted pregnancies as a result of poor absorption of the pill have resulted. Certain antibiotics are toxic to the kidney, especially in patients with impaired kidney function. Aminoglycosides and cephalosporins are important in this regard.

What is penicillin and how is it used?

Penicillin was the first antibiotic, and it has an interesting history. In 1929 a London bacteriologist, Alexander Fleming, noticed that the growth of some staphylococci was inhibited by a chance contaminant of the culture plate. This contaminant was a fungus, *Penicillium notatum*, and the action was due to its production of a substance which Fleming named penicillin. Penicillin was later manufactured in quantity by growing the mould on an industrial scale. The original penicillin, benzyl penicillin, is still used and is the treatment of choice for lobar pneumonia, gonorrhoea, syphilis and infections due to the haemolytic streptococcus, varieties of which cause scarlet fever, rheumatic fever and glomerulonephritis. Benzyl penicillin has a relatively short duration of action and has to be given 4 hourly, by injection. It is not active orally. Long-acting injectable penicillins have been made, an example of which is benzathine penicillin, which maintains satisfactory blood levels of penicillin for up to 3 weeks after a single injection.

The next variety of penicillins developed were the orally active penicillins. These have an action similar to benzyl penicillin but they are not broken down by the acid of the stomach. There are several different varieties, the most well known of which is called penicillin V or phenoxymethyl penicillin. All the drugs have the same limited antibacterial spectrum as the original drug, but semi-synthetic penicillins are now available with a broader spectrum of action. The next innovation was a penicillin not broken down by penicillinase. Present examples are cloxacillin and flucloxacillin. Another innovation were the penicillins with a still wider spectrum of activity, including activity against salmonelli, the bacteria causing enteritis, *Escherichia coli* and *Haemophilus influenzae*. Ampicillin was the first of these compounds, but it has been superceded by amoxycillin which has a similar spectrum but which is better absorbed from the gut than ampicillin. Talampicillin and pivampicillin are also ampicillin-like drugs which produce better blood levels of ampicillin than the original substance. Carbenicillin is a semi-synthetic penicillin which is effective against *Pseudomonas aeruginosa*, a bacterium responsible for certain hospital cross-infections which are extremely difficult to treat.

The penicillins are remarkably safe substances. Their main disadvantage is that patients become allergic to them and an allergic skin rash is quite common. Ampicillin is particularly likely to cause rashes in patients with infectious mononucleosis (glandular fever). In one situation penicillins can be particularly toxic; occasionally in the treatment of meningitis antibiotics are given directly into the CSF through a lumbar puncture needle. With a penicillin this is extremely dangerous. Neural tissue is easily damaged by penicillins and if the drug must be given into the CSF, a special preparation with a low concentration of the drug should be used.

What antibiotics can be used in someone allergic to penicillin?

The general rule is that if a patient is allergic to any of the penicillins, he will be allergic to all of them. Furthermore, patients must be assumed to be allergic to cephalosporins as well. The usual substitutes are erythromycin and tetracycline. Both drugs are absorbed by mouth and are effective against a wide range of organisms.

What are cephalosporins?

The cephalosporins are a group of second-line antibiotics, meaning they are only used when other drugs fail to work. The original cephalosporins had to be given by injection, but there are now oral cephalosporins such as cephalexin, and cephradin. These antibiotics are expensive and sometimes impair kidney function, particularly if given in conjunction with diuretic drugs or to patients with renal failure. Cephalosporins should not be given to patients who are allergic to penicillin.

What are the tetracyclines used for?

Tetracyclines are a widely used group of antibiotics which can be given orally, and are active against a wide range of bacteria. They are particularly useful for treating chronic bronchitis and they are the only effective treatment for rickettsial infections. However, because of their wide antibacterial action, they do cause gastro-intestinal upset and sometimes lead to gut superinfections with yeasts or staphylococci. Another problem is that tetracyclines become incorporated in growing teeth and cause discolouration. For this reason they should not be given to pregnant women or children under the age of 10. Tetracycline should also be avoided in patients with impaired renal function. Date-expired tetracycline tablets can cause renal impairment.

What is the present place of sulphonamides?

Sulphonamides were the first group of antibacterial agents synthesized. The first sulphonamide was a red dye called prontosil, produced in 1935, and it was the first effective treatment for puerperal fever. Sulphonamides are active by mouth. There are some sulphonamides which are poorly absorbed from the bowel and are used to treat intestinal infections. One of the problems with the sulphonamides is that they, or their metabolites, can crystallize in urine if a high enough fluid intake is not taken. In general, the sulphonamides have been superceded by the antibiotics but one substance, sulphasalazine, has a unique use in the maintenance therapy of ulcerative colitis where it has been shown to prolong the interval between acute attacks.

What is co-trimoxazole?

Co-trimoxazole is a mixture of two substances, a long-acting sulphonamide and trimethoprim, a recently discovered substance which interferes with folic acid metabolism. This combination of drugs is particularly effective as it attacks folic acid metabolism in bacteria at two separate points. Co-trimoxazole has been found to be a successful treatment for many different infections, particularly chronic bronchitis and urinary tract infections.

5

Tuberculosis and tropical diseases

What is tuberculosis?

Tuberculosis is a chronic bacterial disease caused by *Mycobacterium tuberculosis.* Usually the infection develops slowly and the illness is prolonged. Any organ in the body can be involved and the clinical signs of the disease are very variable. Although mortality from tuberculosis has fallen steadily in the last century, the disease is still important especially in developing countries and in immigrants from these countries.

Why is tuberculosis different from other bacterial infections?

Tuberculosis is different because of its chronicity, and because the damage caused by the disease is less a result of bacterial invasion than a result of the body's own attempts to react to the organism provoking scar tissue and necrosis. Exposure to tuberculosis is very widespread but only a small proportion of people exposed develop the disease, which is thought to result from a shift in the delicate balance between their immune resistance to tuberculosis and the invasive tendency of the organism.

What forms of tuberculosis are there?

Two stages of disease are recognized, primary tuberculosis and adult tuberculosis. In primary tuberculosis the bacilli infect a previously unexposed individual. The bacilli are rapidly walled off as the specific immunity to the organism is developed. In post-primary or adult tuberculosis specific immunity breaks down and the organism begins to invade the body. Post-primary tuberculosis can result from a new infection or activation of the old primary infection even years after this has been contracted. The two forms of the disease are so different, they were originally thought to be separate illnesses.

How is tuberculosis treated?

Prior to 1940 the treatment of tuberculosis relied on bolstering the patient's resistance with a nutritious diet and sanatorium treatment. Surgical measures were used to promote scarring off of tuberculous lesions. The first drug active against the tubercle bacillus was streptomycin, discovered in 1944. Shortly afterwards *p*-amino salicylic acid (PAS) was introduced and isoniazid, probably the most active of all the anti-tuberculous drugs, was discovered in 1951. Subsequently another six or seven drugs have been added to this list but isoniazid, PAS and streptomycin remain first-line treatment. Even today drug treatment of tuberculosis is a long process lasting a minimum of 6 months, and longer in selected cases.

Why are combinations of drugs used to treat tuberculosis?

Because resistance develops to all anti-tuberculous drugs if they are used singly. Use of a combination of drugs prevents the bacteria from developing a resistant strain. The usual plan is to commence treatment with three drugs, so called triple therapy, and to continue this for 3 months. Triple therapy usually consists of streptomycin, isoniazid and *p*-amino salicylic acid. Streptomycin has to be given by intramuscular injection as it is not absorbed by mouth. Streptomycin also has the disadvantage of being liable to damage the inner ear, causing dizziness and deafness. For patients not in hospital streptomycin must be given during clinic visits twice a week, or the regime can be altered so that two oral drugs can be continued. Unfortunately, one of the main problems with the treatment of tuberculosis is not the efficacy of the drugs but the willingness of the patients to take them. Patients with tuberculosis are often from disadvantaged social groups, often single men living alone, and unless the drugs are given under supervision compliance lapses and reactivation of the tuberculosis can occur.

What other drugs are used?

Newer second rank drugs include ethambutol, which is usually substituted in patients who cannot tolerate PAS, and rifampicin, an effective anti-tuberculous drug which is rather expensive. Other agents include ethionamide and cycloserine. Such drugs are usually used only in specialist units in patients where one of the main line drugs is contraindicated, or in cases where a resistant strain of tuberculosis bacilli has developed.

Why must the duration of treatment be so long?

It is recommended that all patients with tuberculosis should be treated for between 18 and 24 months. Shorter treatment periods of 3 and 6 months have shown an unacceptably high relapse rate. Extended therapy is necessary because the tubercle bacillus is extremely slow growing.

Is surgical treatment of tuberculosis now completely outmoded?

Virtually. Surgical treatment of tuberculosis still has some role to play, but tuberculosis is a good example of a disease completely revolutionized by drug treatment.

What are tropical diseases?

Tropical disease is a waste basket term for infective illness most commonly seen in tropical countries. A detailed exposition on how these diseases are treated is outside the scope of this book, but it may be of interest to discuss an outline of current treatment for some of these illnesses.

How is malaria treated?

As every schoolboy knows, malaria is transmitted by mosquitoes, and anyone entering a malarial area should take prophylactic drugs. In order to be effective these drugs must be taken 24 hours before entering the area and for one month after leaving it. The usual suppressant drugs used as prophylactics are pyrimethamine and proguanil. Once a patient has developed symptomatic malaria the disease can be controlled with a quinine-like agent but complete eradication of the disease can only be achieved using a combination of a quinine-like drug and another agent which is capable of killing the parasite inside the liver.

What other tropical diseases respond to chemotherapy?

Amoebiasis is an infectious disease of the bowel and liver which is frequently seen in patients who have contracted the disease in the tropics. The treatment has been improved considerably in recent years by the use of metronidazole, an antibiotic originally introduced for the treatment of trichomoniasis infections. As is often the case, this drug, originally introduced into clinical medicine for one indication has been found useful in many other diseases, attacking amoebae and a range of anaerobic bacteria.

Cholera is a severe infective diarrhoeal disease where fluid is lost from the bowel in high quantities, up to 20 litres per day. Death is due to dehydration and salt loss. The primary treatment is rehydration with oral salt solutions or with intravenous fluids. Tetracycline is effective against the organism and reduces the bowel loss.

Schistosomiasis is an infestation with the blood fluke, of which there are several species. The main organs affected by this disease are the bladder, the liver and the gut. The disease is a chronic one causing disability by tissue scarring and blood loss. Schistosomiasis is very prevalent in the tropics and is of considerable economic and social importance. Unfortunately, the chemotherapy for this disease is unsatisfactory, being based on antimony containing drugs which have an inherent toxicity. Prevention of re-infection is a major public health problem and the disease will probably not be effectively controlled unless proper sewage systems are installed in endemic areas.

What is the treatment of leprosy?

Contrary to popular belief leprosy is not a very infective illness. The causative organism is an extremely slow growing bacteria with certain affinities to the tubercle bacillus. Drugs are now effective against leprosy but again the treatment must be prolonged in order to be effective. The principal drugs are the dapsones, clofazimine and rifampicin.

6

Drugs and the immune system

What types of treatment affect the immune system?

The immune system of the body is the deliberate target for several sorts of treatment. Vaccines are used to stimulate immunity. Immunity can be bolstered transiently by injection of antibody, either in sera or globulin extracts. This is called *passive immunity* (p. 40). The immune system can also be weakened by immunosuppressive agents which can be useful in autoimmune diseases and have enabled transplant surgery to be undertaken. The immune system is also important because it mediates a common side-effect of drugs, namely allergy.

How does drug allergy come about?

In allergic drug reactions the patient develops an antibody which reacts with the drug (p. 19). Depending where the antibody has been formed, of it, the reaction itself is different. Once an antibody has been formed, and this only happens in a proportion of individuals probably genetically predisposed to allergy, an allergic reaction will take place whenever the drug is administered. Drug rashes are the commonest sort of allergic reaction and are thought to be due to antibodies situated in lymphocyte cells. The severest reaction, anaphylaxis, consisting of wheezing, collapse and urticaria, is mediated by antibodies on the surface of mast cells. When the drug combines with these antibodies, the mast cells break up releasing histamine. Other allergic reactions occur, for example, drug-induced haemolytic anaemia. Serum sickness is a type of allergic reaction where the manifestations are due to circulating antibody–antigen complexes which become deposited in small blood vessels and produce widespread inflammation.

Can allergy be prevented?

Allergy is an idiosyncratic reaction, that is to say it does not occur in all individuals so it is difficult to predict. However, some individuals, namely those who suffer from hay fever, asthma and eczema, are more likely to develop antibodies than other people. Repeated exposure of an individual to the drug favours the development of allergy, and applying the drug to the skin makes it more likely that an allergic reaction will be produced. Practical precautions which can be taken are to ask patients about previous episodes of allergy before they are given drugs. Some drugs are more likely to cause allergy than others and penicillin is particularly notorious in this regard.

What about desensitization?

It is possible to desensitize allergic individuals, but the process is rather elaborate involving many small subcutaneous injections of the allergen at regular intervals. It is also sometimes hazardous as the allergic reaction can be provoked by the treatment, and the benefits are not very long lasting. Desensitizing patients to drugs is only considered where it is absolutely essential that the patient should go on taking an agent and there is no suitable alternative. Desensitization as a treatment for naturally occurring allergies such as hay fever or asthma is sometimes carried out. Desensitizing vaccines containing various allergens, such as pollen extracts and the extract of house mites, are given subcutaneously in gradually increasing doses. In severe hay fever sufferers, this treatment can mean the difference between a good summer and a bad one for the patient, but it does need to be repeated every year.

What are vaccines?

Vaccines are preparations which protect against infectious disease by stimulating the body to produce antibodies to a particular organism. Vaccines are made from organisms which are rendered as harmless as possible while still stimulating an immune response.

How do vaccines work?

Vaccines work by active immunization, stimulating the patient to respond to antigens or immunogenic proteins in the vaccine. The antibodies formed by the recipient are then available to neutralize infecting organisms which possess these same antigens. The vaccination process is named after vaccinia or cow pox, the infection induced by Jenner in 1796 as protection against smallpox. Prior to this the only way of protecting against smallpox was variolization where smallpox itself was induced by inhaling smallpox crusts. The disease this induced was milder than the naturally acquired one but still sometimes fatal.

What hazards are there in vaccination?

Many vaccines are administered by injection and a local reaction, sore arm, is common. Vaccination often produces a transient reaction of fever, headache and malaise, easily treated by rest and aspirin. More serious reactions are uncommon. An immediate allergic reaction with collapse and wheezing is a rare event. Such anaphylactic shock is an emergency, and best treated with subcutaneous adrenaline and parenteral corticosteroids. Patients should be kept under observation for 10–15 minutes after any vaccination in case such a reaction occurs. Recently 'brain damage' has been attributed to pertussis vaccine in infants. The incidence of such vaccine damage, however, is very low.

What vaccines are routinely given to normal individuals?

Children are usually immunized against polio, tetanus, diphtheria and whooping cough. It used to be routine to vaccinate against smallpox, though at the time of writing no case of smallpox has been identified for more than 12 months, so there is some hope that this disease may now be extinct. The other vaccine which is still routinely used is BCG (bacille Calmette-Guérin), a vaccine against tuberculosis. A recent innovation, and a very useful one, is rubella or German measles vaccine which is given to prepubertal girls. Rubella is a mild infection but if acquired in early pregnancy can damage the unborn child. If all women of childbearing age had been vaccinated, this danger would be avoided.

Are there patients who should not be vaccinated?

Vaccination, like any other treatment, carries both risks and potential benefits. Patients with deficiency of immunity and who are on steroids should not be vaccinated. Smallpox vaccine should not be given to patients with eczema or to patients taking steroids, as these predispose to generalized vaccinia. Patients who have had a significant allergic reaction to previous vaccinations should not be vaccinated.

What is passive immunity?

Passive immunity is a way of producing immediate immunity by injecting antibody to the infecting agent. Such antibodies are formed by immunizing an animal, bleeding it and preparing the antibody from the serum. This sort of serum treatment has fallen into disuse as far as the management of infectious disease is concerned. Serum is a rather hazardous material to inject, being very liable to provoke allergic reactions.

What animal sera are in use today?

Animal based antisera are now rarely used; diphtheria antitoxin and snake bite antisera are occasionally used.

Can antibodies from other patients be used?

Yes, human antibodies can be extracted and used in treatment. For example, human antitetanus immunoglobulin is prepared from a pool of plasma taken from donors who have been immunized against tetanus. This preparation can be used to combat early tetanus in a non-immune patient. Human immunoglobulin solution is a preparation also made from pooled normal plasma. The antibody fraction, the γ-globulin, is extracted. This mixture of normal human antibodies is useful in patients who have congenital agammaglobulinaemia and suffer frequent infections. Being a human protein, immunoglobulin is not as immunogenic as animal antibodies. Human immunoglobulin solution can be used to abort or prevent infectious disease. It has been used in women exposed to rubella in pregnancy and in medical staff who have been exposed to hepatitis virus.

What is anti-D and how is it used?

Anti-D is an antibody to the rhesus blood group factor, which is prepared from the blood of rhesus negative individuals who have been immunized against rhesus factor. The antibody is used to prevent a rhesus negative mother from forming antibodies to fetal rhesus positive blood cells. Such fetal cells can get into the maternal circulation during delivery or abortion. The introduction of this treatment is a major advance and if widely applied it could eliminate rhesus baby disease. It is an interesting story; rhesus disease comes about when a woman who has no rhesus antigen on her red blood cells (5% of the population) has a child by a rhesus positive father; the child will be rhesus positive as this is a dominant gene. The mother, if rhesus positive cells from the baby get into her circulation, forms antibodies against the rhesus factor and these antibodies can then attack the baby's cells causing a haemolytic anaemia *in utero*. Usually antibodies are only formed after the first pregnancy so it is the second and subsequent children who are affected. The traditional but hazardous treatment has been to repeatedly transfuse the affected baby *in utero*. Now the disease can be treated by mopping up the fetal cells spilt after birth into the mother's circulation by administering anti-D antibody. In this way the mother is exposed to the antigen only briefly and does not produce antibodies. This treatment can be seen as a brilliant use of immunotherapy and as a triumph of intelligent medicine over cumbersome high technology.

What about serum treatment of snake bites?

This is another example of passive immunization. Snake antivenin is a serum globulin preparation prepared in horses which have been immunized against various snake venoms. The antivenin locally available in different countries varies according to the local snake population. The antivenin is injected intravenously as soon after the bite as possible, and then directly into the bitten area. Severe anaphylactic reactions sometimes occur.

What is immunosuppression used for?

Immunosuppression is a treatment which blunts the immune response. It is employed after transplant surgery to prevent rejection of the foreign organ if it is to function usefully. Immunosuppression is also used where autoimmunity is thought to play a part in the disease process. These diseases include such proven cases as glomerulonephritis where glomerular autoantibodies have been demonstrated, and other diseases where the evidence is less good that autoimmunity plays some role. These include systemic lupus erythematosus, myasthenia gravis and rheumatoid arthritis.

What drugs are used as immunosuppressants?

Three types of drug, corticosteroids, cytotoxics and antilymphocytic serum are used. Corticosteroids in high doses have an immunosuppression action and are frequently used in transplant patients. Cytotoxic drugs include the alkylating agents which work by combining with DNA and upsetting cell division, and antimetabolites which are drugs that combine with enzymes to prevent them working. The most widely used cytotoxic drug used in immunosuppression is azathioprine, but many others are employed including chlorambucil, cyclophosphamide and methotrexate. Antilymphocytic globulin is another example of serum treatment. It consists of globulin from horses immunized to human lymphocytes; these are the cells which mediate one important type of immunity. The purified globulin fraction, lymphocytic antiglobulin, is less toxic than the unpurified serum.

What are the side-effects of immunosuppressants?

Immunosuppression is unfortunately a very toxic treatment. The main hazard is infection to which the immune deficient patient is obviously biased. Even fairly benign infections can produce tremendous reactions in immunosuppressed patients. In addition the high dose steroids have a lot of side-effects, as discussed elsewhere (p. 117). Antilymphocytic globulin treatment has another unsuspected hazard; it apparently predisposes patients to developing tumours, particularly of the lymphoma type.

What drugs are typically used in renal transplant patients?

A typical regime would be large doses of prednisolone, azathioprine, the antibiotic actinomycin C and antilymphocytic globulin.

7

Cancer chemotherapy

What is cancer?

Cancer is the popular term for a malignant neoplasm, and is so called after the Greek for crab. A cancer arises when cells undergo malignant change, escaping the mechanisms which normally hold growth and cell division in check. Tumour cells divide in an unregulated way and spread in the body, both at the site of the original cancer and by remote seeding forming metastases. Tumours of epithelial cells are most common and are called carcinomata. Cancer accounts for about a fifth of deaths in developed countries.

What is the place of drug treatment in malignant disease?

In most cancers the goal of treatment is to cure the patient by removal of the primary tumour before it has spread elsewhere. However, in many patients this is not possible because spread of the tumour has often occurred at the time of diagnosis. Some tumours, such as leukaemia, are by their very nature disseminated at the outset. Drug treatment is the best treatment for some tumours and is a useful adjunct to surgery and radiotherapy in some others.

What is the basis of cancer chemotherapy?

As with antibacterial chemotherapy the principle is to poison the target cells but not the healthy host tissue. Unfortunately, differences between tumour and healthy tissue are slight as they are both derived from the same genetic stock. Some tumour cells divide more rapidly than host cells but this is not invariable. Most anticancer drugs attack cells which are dividing but this does not provide much specificity for the tumour. Cells in the normal gut mucosa and bone marrow also divide rapidly so that these tissues suffer toxicity from the anticancer drugs. Selective biochemical targets in malignant cells are hard to find. Some cancer cells, unlike normal cells, cannot synthesize the amino acid asparagine.

It is thus possible to use this difference therapeutically, by injecting an enzyme, asparaginase, which breaks down asparagine and deprives the tumour of this amino acid. However, this treatment is not very effective and such biochemical differences between tumour and tissue are uncommon. Certain tumours can be influenced by hormonal treatment. Indeed the first successful drug treatment of cancer was when it was discovered that the growth of carcinoma of the prostate could be slowed by estrogen administration.

What cytotoxic drugs are used?

Drugs which kill cells are called *cytotoxics*. Cytotoxic drugs are of various sorts, alkylating agents, antimetabolites, chromosome inhibitors and antibiotics. Radio-active drugs are also used occasionally.

What are alkylating agents?

Alkylating agents are drugs which attack and damage nuclear proteins. They interact with DNA by binding to active groups, chemically transforming the nucleic acid by alkylation. These drugs are the most non-specific of the cytotoxics and include the nitrogen mustards and numerous drugs related to them.

What are antimetabolites?

Antimetabolites are drugs which are analogues of normal metabolites, and act as competitive inhibitors in the cellular processes. In particular they interfere with nucleic acid synthesis. Drugs are known which are inhibitors of purine, pyrimidine and folic acid metabolism. Examples of this group of drugs include 6-mercaptopurine and 5-fluorouracil.

What are chromosome inhibitors?

When chromosomes divide they move to either side of the cell along proteinaceous fibres known as the spindle. Certain drugs are known to bind to this spindle and thus interfere specifically with cell division and are termed *chromosome inhibitors*. These include the alkaloids derived from the periwinkle plant, e.g. vinblastine and vincristine.

What radio-active drugs are used?

Radiation can be applied to a tumour via beams of radiation from an external source, or by implanting radio-active material in the tumour with radium needles or by using a drug which is itself radio-active. Use of this principle is limited by the availability of drugs which will bind directly to tumour tissue. One example is the isotope iodine-131. Iodine is taken up preferentially by the thyroid gland, and ^{131}I is used particularly for the treatment of thyrotoxicosis but it can also be used in the treatment of carcinoma of the thyroid. Another radio-active drug which is used in the treatment of cancer is phosphorus-32. Since phosphorus is concentrated in the bones and in rapidly dividing cells, it can be used to treat polycythaemia vera. Radioactive gold is concentrated in the liver and can be used to treat certain tumours.

What side-effects occur with cytotoxics?

Cytotoxics damage rapidly dividing cells more than slowly growing tissue. Hence their main side-effects are on the bone marrow, producing anaemia and haemorrhage and allowing infection to supervene. In the gut disturbing the growth of the surface epithelium leads to ulceration, haemorrhage, diarrhoea and septicaemia. In the reproductive system such drugs can cause sterility, mutagenesis and teratogenesis. One striking effect of cytotoxic drugs much disliked by patients is hair loss, which occurs due to destruction of the hair follicle; the hair regrows after an interval.

Where are cytotoxic drugs most effective?

Cytotoxic agents are most effective in leukaemia, Hodgkin's disease, lymphomas, prostatic cancer, seminoma and Wilm's tumour. Cure, without recurrence, has been produced in chorion carcinoma, a unique tumour where the cells are partly of fetal origin. The poorest results from chemotherapy are seen in solid tumours such as carcinomas of the cervix and kidney.

How are the drugs used?

Cytotoxic drugs are employed in regimes which have been devised on theoretical grounds, and then validated in clinical trials where one regime is carefully compared with another. The theoretical principles used for devising these regimes are as follows:

(1) To use the maximum tolerated doses of drugs, stopping short of bone marrow failure. In some cases marrow failure may be deliberately induced, and the patient's marrow regenerated after chemotherapy using the patient's own cells which have been collected and stored prior to treatment. A practical point here is that a blood count to assess marrow function is necessary before each new course of cancer chemotherapy.

(2) To use drugs in combination, each having a different mode of action and hence a synergistic effect.

(3) To use supportive regimes of antibiotics, to prevent infection in the patient whose immune system is temporarily suppressed with cytotoxic drugs.

(4) To use drugs together with local radiation therapy, to eradicate the tumour where drugs cannot penetrate, such as the central nervous system.

What hormones are used in cancer?

Corticosteroids are used in the management of many cancers, but are principally useful in blood diseases such as leukaemia. Some neoplastic cells possess highly specific steroid receptors and high doses of steroid can retard their growth. Steroids are also useful in reducing hypercalcaemia produced by metastases to the bone.

Sex hormones are also used in cancer treatment. The beneficial effect of estrogen in cancer of the prostate has been recognized since the 1940s, and the synthetic estrogen, stilboestrol, is still the treatment of choice for disseminated carcinoma of the prostate. Androgens are occasionally used in the treatment of metastatic breast cancer.

When are local infusions of anticancer drugs used?

In an attempt to increase the selectivity of cytotoxic therapy various regimes have been devised to perfuse or infuse the drug directly into the tumour. This is possible when the tumour is peripherally situated, for example in a limb. Local infusion of cytotoxic drugs is also commonly carried out in patients with malignant effusion situated either in the pleural, pericardial or abdominal cavities. Such local treatment with an alkylating agent or antibiotic is a palliative procedure, but it may retard the reaccumulation of the effusion and improve the patient's local symptoms.

What other drugs are used in the treatment of cancer?

Apart from cytotoxic drugs and hormones designed to modify tumour growth, certain other drugs are commonly used. Allopurinol is a drug which prevents the synthesis of uric acid and hence prevents gout. It is commonly used together with cytotoxic drugs, because when large numbers of cells are killed in the body by cytotoxic drugs the quantity of nuclear protein released can lead to a rapid rise in uric acid, hence gout. Another common side-effect of anticancer treatment is nausea and vomiting. This can be treated symptomatically with phenothiazine drugs. Another useful drug is metoclopramide which has been shown to reduce nausea and vomiting if given before a radiation dose.

Are there different types of cytotoxics?

Some cytotoxics are said to be cycle specific and some are called phase specific. Phase specific drugs such as the vinca alkaloids, methotrexate, 6-mercaptopurine and cytosine arabinoside act at specific phases of cell division, and thus affect only the cells at that particular stage of their reproductive cycle. Hence above a certain threshold dose they do not have any addictive effect, having killed all the cells in that particular phase. Other cytotoxic drugs are cell cycle specific, a misleading phrase, which means that they kill cells at all stages of replication. With these drugs there is a dose-response relationship: the greater the dose the greater the toxicity. Because these drugs act differently they can be used with benefit in combination. Cycle specific drugs include cyclophosphamide, doxorubicin and mustine.

SECTION 3

THE CENTRAL NERVOUS SYSTEM

8

Drugs and the central nervous system

How does the brain function?

The brain is a vast collection of excitable nerve cells called neurones separated by a mass of supporting cells called glial cells. Each neurone has a cell body and a large number of cell processes, which reach out to 'connect' with other nerve cells in the brain and other cells outside the central nervous system. A good deal is known about how individual nerve cell function because they can be studied in the peripheral nervous system, and in the primitive nervous systems of invertebrate animals, e.g. squid where there are only a few cells in simple arrangement. The 'connections' between nerve cells are not electrical but chemical. Neurones are excited to transmit electrical stimuli when specialized receptor areas on their cell surfaces are stimulated by a specific neurotransmitter released by another nerve cell. Both inhibitory and excitory neurotransmitters have been identified, and the state of excitation of any given nerve cell is thought to depend on the balance of inhibition and excitation at the many thousands of different interconnections or synapses on the neuronal surface. At individual synapses the rate of release and disposal of the different neurotransmitters is critical. The firing of an individual neurone is complex enough, but each neurone makes only a tiny contribution to the overall activity of the whole organ. How the integration of activity takes place is largely unknown, although the analogy of a huge computer is an attractive one. For the simpler functions, like control of body movement pathways have been defined and a lot is known about them, at least anatomically. However, when more complex functions such as thinking or memory are considered, it must be admitted that we are almost totally ignorant as to how these functions are conducted. Is a memory stored in the brain as a complex molecule, a sophisticated version of a knot in a handkerchief, or is it stored as an electrical charge in an individual nerve cell? We simply do not know the answer to these very basic questions.

What drugs act on the central nervous system?

The drugs whose main site of action is within the brain and spinal cord are among the most widely used in clinical medicine. The drugs include general anaesthetics, narcotic analgesics, hypnotics, sedatives, tranquillizers, antipsychotics, anticonvulsants and drugs used in Parkinson's disease. In addition, those drugs which are used socially, including caffeine and nicotine, all have their action within the central nervous system as do those weapons known as nerve gases.

How do drugs act on the brain?

The action of many centrally acting drugs can be explained in terms of their actions on synaptic activity, usually involving neurotransmitter function in some way. Hence drugs are known which will inhibit release of neurotransmitters, increase synthesis of neurotransmitters, inhibit disposal or metabolism of the neurotransmitter once it is released, or directly attach to the neurotransmitter receptor thereby stimulating or blocking it.

Although most centrally acting drugs appear to work in this way, some do not. The general anaesthetics probably act by a different mechanism, depressing excitation of all nerve cells in the brain by altering the surface membrane excitability of all neurones.

What central neurotransmitters are there?

About a dozen different substances have been identified in the brain, which are thought to act as neurotransmitters. The fact that there are such a small number implies that most of the subtlety of brain function depends on the way in which the synapses are organized. Because of this it is difficult for the pharmacologist to produce drugs having specific actions within the brain, as any drug which affects one neurotransmitter system will affect many millions of different synapses, which may be concerned with completely different functions.

Noradrenaline is a neurotransmitter found in central pathways particularly concerned with mood and arterial blood pressure regulation. Drugs which increase noradrenaline persistence at synapses are used as antidepressants, and drugs which stimulate certain noradrenaline receptors in the hindbrain are used as antihypertensives.

Dopamine has been identified as a neurotransmitter in the nigrostriatal pathway, which has been identified as the nerve tract which degenerates in patients who have Parkinson's disease. Dopaminergic pathways are also concerned with the release of prolactin and are somehow involved with the derangements in psychosis. The major tranquillizers, which are used to treat schizophrenia, act on dopamine receptors.

Serotonin (5-hydroxytryptamine) and histamine are both neurotransmitters within the central nervous system, but their particular function is obscure. Drugs which affect serotonin and histamine receptors have sedative actions but this is probably a non-specific effect.

Acetylcholine is another substance which is almost certainly a neurotransmitter in many central synapses. It is very widely distributed. Atropine-like drugs, which block the effect of acetylcholine at some central synapses are used in the treatment of Parkinson's disease.

Another important set of neurotransmitters are the inhibitory amino acids such as gamma-amino-butyric acid (GABA) and glycine. The actions of benzodiazepine tranquillizers is thought to mimic the effect of GABA on central synapses.

Prostaglandins are also widely distributed in the central nervous system and receptors on nerve cells have been identified which can be stimulated by prostacyclin, one of the more recently discovered prostaglandins.

9

Anaesthetics

What comprises a general anaesthetic?

A typical general anaesthetic consists of a premedication, an induction and an inhalational anaesthetic. Premedication is given to the patient in the ward before being brought to the operating theatre. Anaesthesia is induced by the anaesthetist giving a slow intravenous injection of a short acting anaesthetic agent such as thiopental or methohexitone. This induces a rapid loss of consciousness. The anaesthetic is then maintained by administering a mixture of anaesthetic gases, the active agent being one of the halogenated gases such as halothane or methoxyflurane. The carrier gases include oxygen and nitrous oxide, which is itself a weak anaesthetic. The gas mixture can be administered by face mask or via an intratracheal tube. The patient may either be allowed to breathe the gas mixture spontaneously or artificial ventilation can be used, in which case it is usual to paralyse all the patient's voluntary muscles with a muscle relaxant.

Other drugs and fluids can be administered, as necessary, during the course of the anaesthetic via an intravenous infusion line. When surgery is completed anaesthesia is reversed by stopping all the gases except the oxygen. Muscle paralysis can be reversed by giving a drug antagonist to the muscle relaxant and the patient is extubated. At this point the patient should begin to breathe spontaneously, although remaining difficult to rouse. Post-operative pain can be relieved by intramuscular injections of a narcotic analgesic.

How is a patient prepared for an anaesthetic?

Patients undergoing elective, or planned surgery are often admitted to hospital a day or so prior to operation, so that preliminary steps such as cross matching of blood can be carried out. In addition, their fitness for operation can be confirmed by physical examination or by specialized tests. It is usual for the anaesthetist to visit the patient to assess their condition. Chest infections are a major problem following anaesthesia, and any patient who has evidence of chest infection, cough or head cold should not receive an elective anaesthetic until the infection has been resolved. Immediately before an operation a patient is usually apprehensive and tactful reassurance from the nursing and medical staff is an important part of care. On the day of operation patients are fasted so that they have an empty stomach before going into the theatre. This is a precaution against vomiting during anaesthesia. If a patient inhales vomit into the lungs when their defensive reflexes are depressed by anaesthesia the consequence can be fatal pneumonia.

Why is a premedication often used?

The purpose of the premedication is twofold: to allay the patient's anxiety, thereby making him more amenable during induction of anaesthesia and secondly to reduce bronchial secretion.

What drugs are used as premedications?

A huge variety of drugs are used as premedicants. Most commonly, an anticholinergic drug such as atropine or hyoscine is used. These drugs dry up bronchial secretions and also cause some mental clouding, 'twilight sleep', which is all to the good. Unfortunately, these drugs cause an unpleasantly dry mouth and accelerate the pulse by blocking vagal tone. For these reasons some anaesthetists question their value in a modern anaesthetic and do not use anticholinergics as premedicants.

The other types of drugs used as premedications are sedatives or anxiolytics. Most commonly an opiate narcotic analgesic is used, such as pethidine or papaveretum. Alternatively, a phenothiazine tranquillizer such as promazine or chlopromazine can be used, or even a benzodiazepine such as diazepam. Benzodiazepines produce partial retrograde amnesia. This can be an advantage because details of the operation preparations cannot be remembered by the patient.

How is anaesthesia induced?

Anaesthesia is usually induced with an intravenous injection of a short acting agent such as thiopental or methohexitone. It is possible to induce anaesthesia with an anaesthetic gas administered via a face mask. However, gas induction is rather unpleasant for the patient and may induce confused struggling before anaesthesia is completely established.

Why are muscle relaxants often used in general anaesthesia?

There are two reasons for using muscle relaxants. The first is to make access to the operation site easier for the surgeon as relaxed muscles can be more easily retracted. This is particularly important in abdominal surgery. The second reason is that artificial ventilation is readily carried out if the patient does not 'fight the pump'. One disadvantage of muscle relaxants is that they mask the signs of lightening anaesthesia. When the anaesthesia lightens and the patient begins to sense pain, the first response is tightening of the muscles and some struggling although the patient remains unconscious. If the patient is paralysed with muscle relaxants, obviously no such signs can be seen. It is indeed perfectly possible for a patient given a muscle relaxant to be totally conscious throughout a painful operation if the anaesthetic is not properly administered.

What are muscle relaxants and how do they work?

Muscle relaxants are drugs which paralyse the voluntary muscles. There are two different sorts of drug. The most commonly used is derived from curare, a plant poison used by South American Indians to tip their arrows. Curare blocks the link between motor nerve and voluntary muscle, by competitive antagonism of the neurotransmitter. With normal muscle contraction acetylcholine is released from the nerve and depolarizes the muscle fibre causing it to contract. Curare-like drugs are competitive antagonists, binding to the acetylcholine receptors on the voluntary muscle. The muscle fibre is not depolarized when these receptors are occupied by curare. Curare-like drugs, e.g. tubocurarine, pancuronium or gallamine have a long duration of action after a single intravenous dose, but their effect can be rapidly reversed by injection of an anticholinesterase drug such as neostigmine. Anticholinesterases prevent the normal breakdown of acetylcholine by the enzyme cholinesterase. This results in a build up of acetylcholine and reversal of the curare effect. Curare-like muscle relaxants are used in most lengthy surgical operations.

There is another type of muscle relaxant, the depolarizing muscle relaxants of which suxamethonium is the best example. These drugs work differently. Suxamethonium also binds to the acetylcholine receptor on muscle but causes a prolonged depolarization of the muscle. Its duration of action is rather short, about 5 minutes after each dose, so it is only used to provide muscle relaxation while the trachea is being intubated. The effect of suxamethonium is short lived because it is metabolized by the enzyme pseudocholinesterase which is present in blood. Because suxamethonium causes depolarization of the muscle fibre, the muscles contract transiently. A consequence of this is that post-operative patients receiving suxamethonium often complain of widespread aching muscles, and for this reason suxamethonium is tending to be displaced by the non-depolarizing relaxants. There is no specific antidote to suxamethonium and a small proportion of patients have a deficiency of pseudocholinesterase. In these individuals the paralysis may persist for several hours.

Why are many patients intubated for general anaesthesia?

The purpose of passing an endotracheal tube is primarily to provide a secure airway for the patient during surgery. Obviously if a muscle relaxant is to be given, artificial ventilation then becomes necessary, and it is virtually impossible to perform this efficiently without an endotracheal tube. In patients treated with a muscle relaxant not only is breathing stopped but the jaw and tongue muscles relax, causing the tongue to flop back into the throat and obstruct the airway.

What gases are used in anaesthetics?

All inhalational anaesthetics consist of oxygen, plus one or more anaesthetic agents. It is usual for the mixture to contain nitrous oxide. This gas is a weak anaesthetic but a powerful analgesic agent, and is almost completely non-toxic. Therefore it is a useful carrier gas and can be employed for short anaesthetics as in dentistry. However, most of the anaesthetic effect of modern inhalational anaesthetics is produced by one or other of the halogenated anaesthetic gases, halothane being the most commonly used. Introduced in 1956, it is a sweet smelling and potent anaesthetic in an inhalational dose of 1–3% of the inhaled gases. One of its important additional effects is to cause dilatation of blood vessels and a consequent fall in blood pressure, probably because the central nervous system maintains the tone of blood vessels via the autonomic nervous system, and depression of central centres leads to loss of this control. In very deep anaesthesia or anaesthetic overdose a profound fall in blood pressure occurs. Halothane is a safe anaesthetic but should be avoided if repeated anaesthetics are required, because in these circumstances it can cause jaundice and liver damage.

Alternative gases include methoxyflurane and enflurane. These gases have virtually displaced anaesthetic ether, because they are safe and non-inflammable while ether can explode if exposed to electrical sparks or high temperature diathermy.

How do gaseous anaesthetics work?

The precise mechanism of action of general anaesthetics is not known. Various suggestions have been put forward, one of the most likely being that general anaesthetics act as organic solvents disrupting important cell surface phenomena in nerve cells and so depressing nervous excitability.

What are the hazards of gaseous anaesthetics?

Modern general anaesthesia is a remarkably safe procedure. Most of the risk lies not in adverse effects of the anaesthetic drugs but in mechanical errors in administering the anaesthetic gases. Hypoxia or anoxia due to mechanical failure of the anaesthetic system, mixing up the gases, or failure to secure an effective airway are by far the most important hazards.

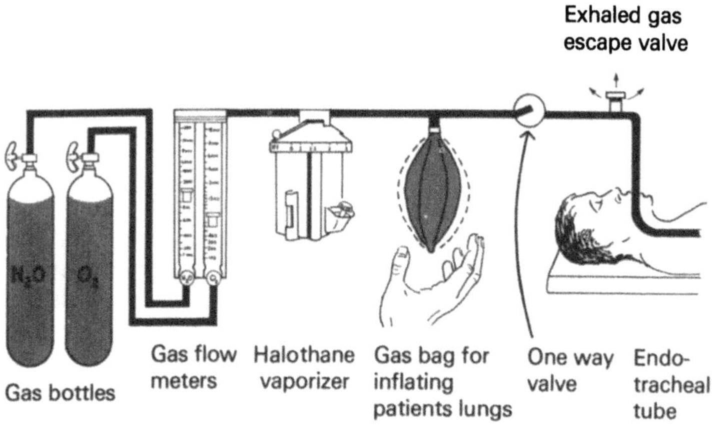

Figure 4 Components of an open circuit anaesthetic apparatus for giving an anaesthetizing mixture of oxygen, nitrous oxide and halothane

How does an anaesthetic machine work?

An anaesthetic machine looks complicated but it is essentially extremely simple (Figure 4). It consists of a source of oxygen under pressure, usually a cylinder with a valve and flow meter. Similarly, there is a source of nitrous oxide with a valve and flow meter. A volatile halogenated anaesthetic such as halothane is added to this gas mixture by bubbling the gas through a vaporizer. This is so designed that the amount of halothane added can be simply adjusted by turning a dial on the vaporizer. The mixture of anaesthetic gases so produced is then led to the patient. The patient breathes in the anaesthetic gas mixture from the machine, and out into the theatre atmosphere through a non-return valve. This is the so-called 'open circuit'. However, it is also possible to have a closed circuit machine, in which the patient's exhaled gases re-enter the machine and carbon dioxide is absorbed by soda lime. More oxygen is added and the mixture rebreathed. A final sophistication in modern equipment is the incorporation of a respirator, which blows the anaesthetic gas mixture into the patient at the required frequency and pressure to produce artificial ventilation.

What are the stages of anaesthesia?

Early in the history of anaesthesia it was noticed that as the patients sank into deepening anaesthesia their behaviour changed. These changes were described as different stages of anaesthesia and were a help in gauging the level of anaesthesia during the administration of some of the crude early anaesthetics. In modern practice this staging has largely been discarded because the changes are masked by muscle relaxants. Stage I is where the patient is still conscious but has a reduced perception of pain. Stage II is where the patient is unconscious but is active, irrational and excitable. Stage III is the deeper stage of full anaesthesia when the active struggling of Stage II has ceased.

10

Analgesics

What is an analgesic?

An analgesic is a drug used to relieve pain. There are two sorts of analgesics, narcotic analgesics and minor analgesics. Narcotics relieve pain by an action within the central nervous system and their use is restricted because they can cause addiction. Minor analgesics act in a completely different way, suppressing pain and inflammation by a local action in the tissue concerned. They are not addictive.

What are narcotic analgesics used for?

Narcotics are the most effective drugs for severe pain but because of the addiction problem, their use is restricted to occasions whether either the pain is likely to be temporary, as after surgery, or uncontrollable by other measures as in the pain of terminal cancer. Narcotic analgesics are especially useful in myocardial infarction because they both relieve the distress of the pain and produce vasodilatation, aiding the compromised heart. Apart from relieving pain and producing vasodilatation, narcotics have two other actions which are useful clinically: inhibition of gut peristalsis and suppression of cough. Hence weak mixtures of narcotics such as kaolin and morphine are useful in the relief of diarrhoea, and narcotics of the codeine type are the basis of many cough mixtures.

What narcotic drugs are there?

There are many narcotics. Some are still prepared from the opium poppy while others are entirely synthetic. They differ both in their potency and tendency to induce dependence. On this basis the narcotics can be roughly divided into two groups. Morphine, heroin, methadone, pethidine and pentazocine are powerful analgesics and have an appreciable tendency to induce addiction. Codeine, dihydrocodeine, and dextropropoxyphene are less powerful analgesics with little tendency to induce addiction. As a result, these drugs are more freely used for trivial conditions and as cough suppressants.

What actions and side-effects does morphine have?

Morphine is usually given by injection because its absorption by mouth is irregular. A 10–15 mg dose of morphine relieves pain within 15 minutes of administration, and the effects last for 3–4 hours, the action of the drug being terminated when it is metabolized in the liver and excreted in the urine. The pain relief after morphine is dissociative. This means that the pain is still felt but the patient becomes indifferent to it. Morphine has a euphoric action, making the patient more cheerful; it also sedates the patient and induces sleep. All these are desirable effects in an exhausted patient with severe pain, but undesirable effects also occur, respiratory depression, tolerance and addiction being the most serious. A proportion of patients are nauseated when given morphine and it is often administered together with an antiemetic such as cyclizine to overcome this problem. Morphine depresses respiration and for this reason can be dangerous in patients with lung disease whose respiratory reserve is impaired. Morphine also induces constipation and constriction of the pupils. Pinpoint pupils are a characteristic sign of opiate administration.

Overdosage with morphine can be fatal. The patient is usually unconscious, cyanosed and sweating. Pinpoint pupils, depressed respiration, slow pulse and low blood pressure are characteristic. Since repeated doses of morphine cause tolerance to its effects, morphine addicts can take large doses of the drug without signs of overdosage. Conversely, patients with impaired liver function, who are unable to metabolize the drug rapidly, can show overdosage symptoms from normal sized doses. Morphine should not be given to children under 1 year of age, as their livers are not mature enough to metabolize the drug.

What does narcotic addiction consist of?

Narcotic addiction is associated with tolerance to the effect of repeated doses of narcotics, a craving for repeated administration and the occurrence of withdrawal symptoms when the drug is stopped. Physical dependence only occurs after treatment for 1–2 weeks, and contrary to popular opinion cannot occur after a single dose. Withdrawal symptoms include yawning, sneezing, a running nose, tremor, sweating, anxiety, restlessness, nausea, vomiting and diarrhoea. Withdrawal of drug from narcotic addicts is best accomplished gradually, substituting decreasing doses of methadone for the opiate being used. Opiate addiction has both a social and a pharmacological basis. In fact the opiate habit is easier to give up than is cigarette smoking; rates of relapse are much higher in patients trying to give up cigarettes than they are in addicts who genuinely wish to give up narcotics.

How do narcotic analgesics work?

Natural morphine-like substances called endorphins are found in the brain, and neuronal receptors for these substances have been identified. Narcotics stimulate these receptors. The normal function of the natural morphine-like system in the brain is thought to be concerned with appreciation of satisfaction and pleasure. It is interesting that activation of this euphoriant system is provoked by stress. It seems that appreciation of pain can be suppressed briefly if a life-threatening situation arises. The mechanism allows evasive action to be taken even if the individual is injured and would normally be immobilized by pain. Such a system would have an obvious survival value and opiate drugs artificially activate the system.

It is certainly curious that many plants contain drugs which can specifically activate receptors in mammalian tissue. The occurrence of opium alkaloids in poppy heads is a classic example of this extraordinary phenomenon; another example is the presence of nicotine in tobacco.

What about other narcotics?

Heroin is very similar to morphine, but for an equal analgesic effect the euphoria is greater and the gastro-intestinal side-effects less. For these reasons heroin is the preferred drug of narcotic addicts, and indeed its medical use is, for this reason, forbidden in the USA. In the UK heroin is used as the drug of choice in myocardial infarction and in left ventricular failure.

Methadone is a less sedative analgesic than morphine, is more consistently absorbed by mouth and has a less euphoric effect. Its main use is in the oral treatment of severe pain and in withdrawal programmes for drug addicts.

Pethidine is a synthetic opiate frequently used for post-operative pain and in labour. It is less sedative than morphine and has a shorter effect of 2–3 hours.

Pentazocine is another synthetic opiate and of the powerful analgesics has the least tendency to induce dependence. It is also consistently effective when given orally.

Codeine, dihydrocodeine, and dextropropoxyphene are all narcotic analgesics with a low addiction potential, and are also less powerful analgesics than morphine. Codeine is frequently used for the relief of mild to moderate pain, and codeine linctus is one of the best treatments for an unproductive cough.

Can the effects of the narcotics be reversed?

Reversal of opiate effects can be produced by naloxone, a competitive antagonist of morphine, and which has no analgesic effects of its own. This drug is used in the treatment of opiate overdose, and to treat neonates who have respiratory depression following transfer of a narcotic across the placenta during labour. It is interesting that naloxone can reverse the analgesic effect of placebo injection, suggesting that the placebo effect involves activation of the endogenous endorphin system.

What are minor analgesics and how do they work?

Over the years many drugs with mild analgesic actions have been discovered. Aspirin and paracetamol are the most well known and many others such as indomethacin, phenylbutazone and ibuprofen have a similar range of effects, i.e. reducing inflammation and fever and relieving pain. In the early 1970s it was discovered that all these drugs had one biochemical action in common, inhibition of the formation of prostaglandins. This is now thought to be their mode of action.

What are prostaglandins?

Prostaglandins are substances derived from fatty acids and appear to be formed in all animal cells. There are a large number of them and they have many different actions. Prostaglandins appear to be particularly important in inflammation; they are released when tissue is damaged and cause an increase in blood flow through the tissue and stimulate sensory nerve endings causing pain. Release of prostaglandins in the brain is thought to be an important step in the elevation of body temperature in fever. Aspirin-like drugs, also known as minor analgesics or non-steroidal anti-inflammatory drugs (NSAID), inhibit cyclo-oxygenase, the principal enzyme responsible for synthesizing prostaglandins in tissue. Inhibition of prostaglandin formation interferes with the mechanisms of inflammation, pain and fever.

Aspirin-like drugs inhibit other enzymes to a greater or lesser extent, and these additional effects probably account for the different clinical usefulness of the different drugs. For example, some drugs inhibit the lipoxygenase enzyme which synthesizes substances principally concerned with attracting inflammatory cells into damaged tissue. Drugs such as benoxaprofen which inhibit this enzyme have a particularly strong anti-inflammatory effect.

How can analgesics help in treating arthritis?

Minor analgesics are the mainstay of treatment for the main forms of arthritis, osteoarthritis and rheumatoid arthritis. However, these drugs provide only symptomatic relief of pain and inflammation and do not modify the underlying disease process. In severe arthritis corticosteroids have a place in treatment either systemically or by direct injection into the joint. Other drugs used in arthritis include penicillamine and gold salts. Both are toxic drugs and it is doubtful if they really alter progression of arthritis.

What side-effects do the mild analgesics produce?

By far the most important is the tendency of all these drugs to cause gastric bleeding. Patients on continuous treatment with aspirin lose small amounts of blood into the gut and may become anaemic. Sometimes frank ulceration of the stomach occurs with haematemesis and melaena.

11

Hypnotics

What is an hypnotic?

An hypnotic is a drug which induces sleep; the term is really synonomous with sedative. Hypnotics are among the most frequently prescribed drugs and 'sleeping pills' are one of the greatest boons or greatest evils of our time, depending on one's point of view. The real problem with drug-induced sleep is that it is not identical to natural sleep. In natural sleep a series of physiological cycles occur; on falling asleep one enters a phase of relaxed deep sleep, but at intervals this changes abruptly to a more wakeful phase of sleep known as rapid eye movement sleep (REM). REM sleep periods last up to 20 minutes and during this time the sleeper moves his limbs and his eyes and experiences dreams. REM sleep is probably an important restorative component of sleep, and hypnotics tend to suppress this phase, inducing prolonged deep sleep which may not be as refreshing.

When should hypnotics be prescribed?

The use of a drug to combat insomnia is justified, provided that the drug usage will be temporary and not indefinitely prolonged. The legitimate use of hypnotics is to help a patient through a period of grief or anxiety when sleep is difficult. The problem is that patients become accustomed to using these drugs and become dependent upon them.

What hypnotics are there?

Many different cerebral depressants induce sleep, and sedation is a relatively non-specific side-effect of many drugs such as tranquillizers, centrally acting antihypertensives, antidepressants and so on. The drugs most often used as sleeping tablets are the benzodiazepines, but barbiturates, chlorals and methaqualone are also used.

What are the main problems with hypnotic drugs?

Apart from suppressing REM sleep, hypnotics have a variety of side-effects:

(1) Hangover. On waking next day, some carry-over of the sedative effect of the hypnotic drug is inevitable if an effective dose of drug is taken. Even when the patient is not aware of being sedated, careful tests of alertness can detect this hangover effect even in the afternoon following the drug dosage.

(2) Habituation. There is a tendency with all these drugs for patients to become dependent upon them, and so continue to take them long after the initial indication has ceased, and to experience withdrawal symptoms if the drug is stopped.

(3) Abuse. Hypnotic drugs are amongst the most frequently used in deliberate overdosage and barbiturates alone account for about 25% of all suicide attempts.

(4) Drug interactions. Barbiturates, but not the benzodiazepines, induce the production of extra drug metabolizing capacity in the liver. Hence patients taking these drugs have a speeded-up elimination rate of other drugs normally metabolized in the liver. This can have serious consequences if the dosage of the second drug is not adjusted appropriately. For example, women taking low dosage contraceptive pills can become pregnant if they take barbiturates at the same time.

What are the relative merits of the different drugs used as hypnotics?

Benzodiazepines are in general safer than the other hypnotics. The main advantages of the benzodiazepines is that they have a high therapeutic ratio and hence are unlikely to be fatal, even when they are taken in huge overdosage. This is the most important advantage that they have over barbiturates. However, benzodiazepines taken long term for their hypnotic effect or as anti-anxiety agents can produce psychological and physiological dependence. Psychological dependence is an emotional compulsion to take the drug, and the preoccupation with securing its supply. Physical dependence is characterized by tolerance and by withdrawal symptoms on stopping the drug. These symptoms include agitation, tremor, headache and nausea. However, benzodiazepine dependence is not a great problem. It certainly does not occur in patients treated for a few weeks or so.

What about barbiturates?

The barbiturates are a family of sedative drugs which include drugs useful as anticonvulsants and as anaesthetic agents. The use of barbiturates as sleeping tablets is now outmoded. Barbiturates suppress REM sleep more than the benzodiazepines do, and are dangerous even in moderate overdosage, whereas benzodiazepines are not. Furthermore, dependence on barbiturates is a much more serious problem than it is with the benzodiazepines. Patients who become habituated to barbiturates should have the drugs withdrawn slowly, as severe withdrawal symptoms can occur even leading to epileptic convulsions and death. Benzodiazepines can be substituted in the withdrawal programme.

In addition, barbiturates may be deliberately abused by drug users because they cause elation, distortion of judgement and a sensation of the swift passage of time.

What other sedatives are there?

Chloral hydrate is an unpleasant tasting drug, usually given in solution or in a compound form such as dichloralphenazone. Chloral drugs are traditionally used as sedatives in the elderly and the young. They are effective but probably not in any way superior to small doses of the benzodiazepines. Chlormethiazole and methaqualone are effective sleeping tablets but they have no advantage over the benzodiazepines and have little to recommend them. Both cause physical dependence.

Which benzodiazepine is the best hypnotic?

There are many different benzodiazepines and some of these drugs have been marketed as anxiolytics and others as hypnotics. In fact it is now recognized that all these drugs have identical pharmacological effects, and the only difference between them is their rate of elimination from the body, which in turn depends on their rate of metabolism in the liver. Short-acting benzodiazepines are obviously better suited for use as hypnotic drugs than are the long-acting benzodiazepines, which are ideally suited for use as anxiolytics as their effect is prolonged. The short-acting drugs suitable for use as hypnotics include temazepam, lorazepam and oxazepam. There is little point in changing the patient from one of these drugs to another as each has a similar action and the choice is an arbitrary one.

What other measures can be effective in insomnia?

Obviously any underlying condition should be treated. Some alteration of the patient's sleeping arrangements may be effective; a walk before retiring is a simple pleasure the insomniac should be encouraged to enjoy. The old standby of a milk drink before bed is another simple but effective manoeuvre.

12

Antiepileptics

What is epilepsy?

Epilepsy is a medical condition where convulsions or fits occur, and is a common condition affecting 1 in 200 of the population. There are several different types of epilepsy. In *grand mal* the fit is striking and once seen never forgotten. The patient loses consciousness, goes rigid for a few moments, then jerks repetitively, finally falling into a stuporous sleep. *Petit mal* is a disease of children in which very brief periods of unrousability occur, often many times a day. In *focal epilepsy* the convulsion is localized to one limb or muscle group, and there is usually a localized brain lesion to account for this condition. In *temporal lobe* epilepsy the attack may consist of an intense internal experience or automatic behaviour.

Epilepsy can be caused by head injury, meningitis or cerebral tumour, but in most cases there is no recognizable cause and the disease is *idiopathic*, i.e. 'without cause'.

How can epilepsy be treated?

The only effective treatment of epilepsy is by using anticonvulsant drugs, which can both suppress attacks and abort an epileptic attack as it occurs. Some factors are known which increase the frequency of fits in epileptics. These include exhaustion, intercurrent illness, alcohol, antidepressant drugs and flashing lights. Obviously these must be avoided.

How do anticonvulsant drugs work?

Epileptic fits are thought to occur when the paroxysmal discharge of a group of abnormal neurones spreads to adjacent brain regions. Anticonvulsant drugs reduce the excitability of cerebral neurones and reduce the frequency with which these paroxysms occur. Some drugs also reduce the likelihood of the discharge spreading to other regions of the brain. Several of the newer anticonvulsants are thought to act through the intervention of γ-amino butyric acid (GABA); this is a central neurotransmitter which is thought to normally act as an inhibitor of brain discharges thus reducing repetitive firing of stimulated neurones. Both sodium valproate and the benzodiazepines are thought to act through this system.

When should anticonvulsant drugs be used?

All patients with established active epilepsy should be placed on prophylactic drug therapy designed to minimize fit frequency. Treatment with long term anticonvulsants is the norm in epilepsy. In patients who have had no fits for 3 years, cautious gradual withdrawal of the drug therapy can be attempted.

What are the principles of using anticonvulsant therapy?

It used to be common to use a combination of several different anticonvulsants to treat epilepsy. Recent research indicates that epileptics can be more effectively treated with a single drug, provided that the dosage of the drug is carefully adjusted. This choice of a correct dose for each patient is best achieved by measuring the plasma concentration of the drug after different doses. A single drug is preferable to a combination because one anticonvulsant tends to alter the metabolism of another, and thus it is difficult to optimize the dose of each drug in the presence of another.

What anticonvulsant drugs should be used?

This depends on the type of epilepsy. For grand mal epilepsy either phenytoin, phenobarbitone, carbamazepine or sodium valproate are reasonable choices. For petit mal ethosuximide is the first choice, troxidone the second choice. For temporal lobe epilepsy phenobarbitone or sodium valproate are preferred.

How is phenytoin used?

Phenytoin is a very effective antiepileptic drug, which is less sedative than phenobarbitone. In overdosage phenobarbitone produces unsteadiness of speech and gait, and double vision before it causes drowsiness. Different individuals metabolize phenytoin at different rates and the dose needs to be adjusted for each patient. This is best done by measuring the plasma level of the drug, and adjusting the dosage carefully until the right plasma level (between 10 and 20 μg/ml) is achieved. Below this level fits may not be controlled, and above this level toxic symptoms tend to set in. It is difficult to use phenytoin properly without measuring plasma levels.

Phenytoin is taken once during the evening, a reasonable starting dose being 300 mg. Over the long term, phenytoin has several unfortunate side-effects including coarsening of the facial features and hypertrophy of the gums. In pregnancy it may increase the incidence of cleft palate in the baby. However, the risk of this malformation is still low, about 1 in 20 in women taking phenytoin, and is not sufficient to justify stopping the drug.

What about phenobarbitone?

Phenobarbitone is a barbiturate with a long halflife of about 4 days and hence needs to be taken only once a day. Phenobarbitone is sedative but patients soon become tolerant to this effect. Another anticonvulsant, primidone, is thought to chiefly act by being metabolized to phenobarbitone in the liver. Long term phenobarbitone treatment is generally free of toxicity but osteomalacia and macrocytic anaemia due to folate deficiency can be produced.

What about carbamazepine?

Carbamazepine is a drug chemically related to imipramine with a rather long halflife of around 18 hours. Side-effects are dose related, and as with phenytoin this drug can cause blurred vision and unsteadiness.

What side-effects does sodium valproate have?

Sodium valproate is less sedative than the barbiturates and the most frequent side-effects are nausea and lack of appetite. Some patients develop baldness on this drug.

What about refractory epilepsy?

Patients whose fits persist despite drug treatment should have the diagnosis reviewed to see whether the type of drug is appropriate for the variety of epilepsy they have, and whether they might have some active underlying disease. The concentration of anticonvulsant in their plasma should be measured to see whether the patient is taking the optimum dose of drug. Patients who are not controlled on a single drug and have fits while the plasma concentration is in the therapeutic range should be started on an additional drug.

What about status epilepticus?

Status epilepticus is a dangerous condition where one fit follows another without a return to consciousness. The patient may die or suffer brain damage due to anoxia during the tonic phase of the fit. The fit must be stopped by intravenous drug therapy, the best drug being diazepam, which can if necessary be given by continuous infusion. In severe cases it may be necessary to use a muscle relaxant and to put the patient on a ventilator.

13

Psychotropic drugs

What drugs are available for treating mental disease?

Psychotropic drugs or drugs acting on mental functions are among the most widely prescribed in medicine, and the discovery of drugs with specific actions on mood and thought has been an important recent development which has revolutionized psychiatry. There are three main types of psychotropic drugs, the antipsychotics, the anxiolytics and the antidepressants.

What is psychosis?

The biochemical basis of mental disease remains obscure, so a scientific classification of the various disorders is rather difficult. However mental illness can be divided into two broad classes, psychosis and neurosis. Patients with neurosis have disturbances in mood and feeling but still retain contact with reality. Psychotics show certain characteristic disturbances of thought, which indicate that they are either partly or wholly out of touch with the real world around them.

It has been discovered quite empirically that certain drugs known as antipsychotics or major tranquillizers have a therapeutic effect in psychotic patients, in some cases returning their behaviour to normal. There are two sorts of antipsychotics: phenothiazines and butyrophenones.

What are the effects of phenothiazines?

The major action of the phenothiazine drugs is to produce a state of calm without drowsiness. Chlorpromazine was the first drug of this type and is still the standard. It reduces overactivity, excitement and confusion, and produces a feeling of detachment. It is also useful as an antiemetic.

When it was first introduced chlorpromazine revolutionized the treatment of psychiatric patients, and the widespread use of phenothiazine-like drugs has enabled a large number of psychotic individuals to leave institutional care and take up a semi-normal existence in society. One problem with these individuals is to continue their treatment as out-patients since psychotics often fail to take oral medication. Several types of injectable depot phenothiazines have been developed and can be administered every 2 or 3 weeks to such patients.

What side-effects do phenothiazines produce?

The side-effects of phenothiazines include sedation, hypotension, dry mouth and blurring of vision. Some patients get idiosyncratic toxic effects such as jaundice and some develop Parkinson-like syndromes. This is explicable pharmacologically, these drugs are thought to have their main action by blocking dopamine receptors in the brain and, as is explained in Chapter 14 on Parkinson's disease, dopamine receptors are involved in involuntary movement control.

Another problem with phenothiazine therapy is *tardive dyskinesia.* This is usually only a problem in patients who have taken the drug chronically for a period of years. It consists of involuntary movements, particularly of the mouth. Unfortunately these effects are not reversible and indeed on stopping the drug they become worse. Tardive dyskinesia is a common problem in chronic patients, but fortunately it does not seem to cause the patients themselves much distress.

What about the butyrophenones?

These drugs have pharmacological actions very similar to those of the phenothiazines, although they have a different chemical structure. The most widely used in haloperidol, which is particularly useful in the management of manic confused patients. These drugs are also used in so-called 'neurolept analgesia' because of the feeling of detachment they produce.

What are the anxiolytics?

Anxiolytics are drugs which have a specific tranquillizing effect on anxiety. Unfortunately anxiety is an extremely common symptom, either on its own or associated with other medical conditions. In some patients it can be disabling and treatment is indicated. The drugs used as anxiolytics are known as minor tranquillizers and include the benzodiazepine drugs and benzoctamine. Barbiturates were once used in the treatment of anxiety but their use is now frowned upon because of the suicide risk and problems of habituation.

Which benzodiazepines are used for anxiety?

As previously mentioned all the many benzodiazepines have almost identical pharmacological actions. The only difference between the drugs is their rate of elimination from the body. Benzodiazepines with long halflives are best suited for treating anxious patients since single daily doses are effective. Benzodiazepines with long halflives include diazepam, nitrazepam and chlordiazepoxide. The main difficulty with anti-anxiety agents is that they are very effective and patients become dependent upon their use. Physical dependency can also occur with withdrawal symptoms. However, in other respects these drugs are relatively innocuous, and serious side-effects are extremely uncommon. The mode of action of benzodiazepines is not known but they probably act via GABA, an inhibitory neurotransmitter present throughout the central nervous system. GABA is thought to act as a sort of chemical insulation in the CNS, preventing repetitive firing of neurones and interaction of one neurone with another.

What is depression?

Depression is a condition where profound unhappiness makes the patient miserable and withdrawn. As the patient's life becomes dominated by intolerable feelings of dejection, thought and action may be slowed up and the patient appears retarded and sluggish. Depression precipitated by some unhappy event such as bereavement is termed reactive depression while depression with no obvious cause is termed endogenous.

Is depression a disease?

We are all depressed on occasion. However, in some individuals depression becomes so prolonged, inappropriate and profound that it is obviously pathological. It is as well to remember in this connection that depression may be a fatal disease, and indeed suicide is a very important and usually preventable cause of death. Suicide is most common amongst single people living on their own. The peak ages for suicide are the early 20s and the over 60s.

What is manic depression?

Some individuals show an exaggerated swing of mood from euphoric grandiosity to deep depression. Once again these swings are greatly exaggerated variants of normal swings of mood from which we all suffer. Manic depression in its most florid form is in fact a psychosis and the patients often exhibit features of schizophrenia. The importance of the distinction of manic depression from pure depression is that lithium is the treatment of choice rather than standard antidepressants.

What is lithium?

Lithium is a metal, similar to sodium, which forms salts which can be used for the treatment of mood disturbances. Lithium was first introduced into clinical practice in the mid 1960s, and is now recognized as the standard treatment for mania. Lithium treatment, if it is to be effective, must be taken extremely regularly and plasma levels of lithium must be monitored at intervals. The dose varies with weight, renal clearance, age, fluid intake and sodium levels, and it is extremely important to get the right dose. A deliberate overdose of lithium can be extremely dangerous, producing cardiovascular collapse and prolonged coma. Severely poisoned patients can be managed with haemodialysis.

What about drug treatment of depression?

The rationale for drug treatment of depression is that this represents a disturbance of monoamine metabolism in the brain. The brains of depressed patients show lower concentrations of monoamines in certain regions than those dying from other causes. Drugs which reduce monoamines in the brain can produce depression. Drug therapy is aimed at increasing brain monoamine levels. This can be done by interfering with the active transport mechanism in monoaminergic neurones which terminates the actions of released monoamines. Drugs with such an action are known as tricyclic antidepressants. Another way of achieving the same end is to prevent the breakdown of noradrenaline and serotonin by drugs which inhibit the enzyme monoamine oxidase (MAOI).

What are the tricyclic antidepressants?

Tricyclic antidepressants are the most commonly used antidepressant drugs and include such drugs as imipramine and amitriptyline. There are considerable interindividual differences in the plasma halflives of these drugs, and different individuals can have vastly different steady-state plasma concentrations on the same dose. The halflife of the drugs is long and they can be taken once a day, preferably at night as they have a sedative action. Tricyclic antidepressants take at least 3 weeks to exert any effect, and it is often difficult to get patients who are depressed to persist with the treatment.

What about monoamine oxidase inhibitors?

Monoamine oxidase inhibitors (MAOI) are effective antidepressant drugs but they have one major defect; all the existing drugs require fairly elaborate dietary precautions. The drugs inhibit MAO enzymes in the gut wall as well as in the brain. A consequence of this is that the amine tyramine can be absorbed from food containing it, rather than being destroyed by the enzyme. If tyramine gains access to the circulation it can cause a hypertensive crisis. Because of this patients on MAOI have to eat a special diet where foodstuffs containing tyramine are eliminated. Any food which has fermented contains the amine, so cheese, wine and many vegetables are forbidden.

14

Parkinson's disease

What is Parkinson's disease?

Parkinson's disease or Parkinsonism is a disorder of voluntary movement where the patient shows slowing of voluntary movement, muscular rigidity and tremor. The face of a patient suffering from Parkinsonism is characteristic. They blink infrequently, the eyes have a staring appearance and the face is fixed in a rigid expressionless gaze. In most patients no definite cause for Parkinsonism can be found but it occasionally follows encephalitis, and a similar syndrome can be induced by chronic treatment with certain drugs, particularly the antipsychotics and the antihypertensives reserpine and methyldopa.

What brings about the syndrome?

Parkinsonism is one of the few neurological diseases where we have good insight into the biochemical mechanism. It has been known for a long time that in Parkinson's disease there is a degeneration of the basal ganglia, i.e. cellular masses at the base of the brain. From biochemical measurements of the brains of patients with Parkinsonism and from the therapeutic effects of drugs, it appears that the disorder is one of disturbance of balance between two types of neurone in this area. The first type of neurone is cholinergic, i.e. releasing acetylcholine and the other dopaminergic, i.e. releasing dopamine. In Parkinson's disease the basic lesion is the degeneration of the neurones which produce dopamine, allowing relative overactivity of the cholinergic neurones (Figure 5). The situation is probably much more complicated than this, but it provides a useful scheme for understanding the different drugs used in Parkinsonism.

How is Parkinsonism treated?

Basically there are two different types of drug for treating Parkinson patients; those which act to reduce the effect of the cholinergic neurones, anticholinergic drugs, and those which act in different ways to increase the activity of the failing dopaminergic neurones.

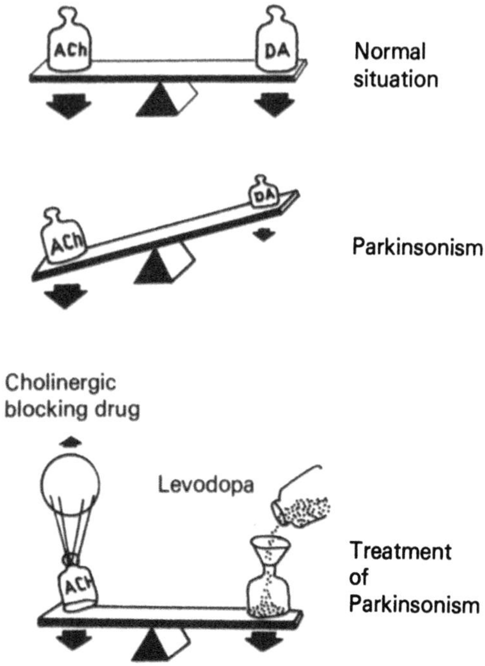

Figure 5 Shows the neurotransmitter imbalance which occurs in Parkinsonism, and how treatment is planned to correct the situation

What anticholinergic drugs are used?

Anticholinergic drugs were first introduced more than 100 years ago by Charcot because they reduce salivation, and dribbling from an immobile mouth is one of the problems in Parkinson's disease. Charcot found, however, that not only was the salivation reduced but the patients' immobility was also helped by belladonna, the atropine-like preparation used at that time. Nowadays, various synthetic anticholinergic drugs are used such as benzhexol, or orphenadrine or benztropine. The drugs are taken in the maximum tolerated dose, i.e. until side-effects such as blurring of vision and dry mouth become pronounced. Unfortunately only about one third of Parkinson's patients derive much benefit from the use of these drugs.

What about dopaminergic drugs?

The use of dopaminergic drugs is relatively recent and has been a major breakthrough in the treatment of Parkinson's disease. The development of these drugs is in fact of considerable interest, because it is one of the few drug treatments which has been designed rationally on the basis of biochemical findings in the brain of patients suffering from the disease. Although the neurones which produce dopamine are depleted in Parkinsonian patients, it is possible to increase their activity by supplying them with an increased amount of the precursor substance which the neurones make into dopamine. This precursor substance is called dopa. One cannot give dopamine itself because it is inactivated by the enzyme monoamine oxidase in the gut when given by mouth. However, L-dopa is absorbed by mouth and can enter the brain and be used by the dopaminergic system to manufacture more dopamine.

Three other types of drug are used which act on the dopaminergic system. Bromocryptine is a drug related to ergot, which has been developed to specifically mimic the effect of dopamine at its receptor. Amantadine is an amine drug which was originally discovered to have an antiparkinsonian action when it was used to treat a flu-like illness in a patient with Parkinson's disease. Amantadine probably works by making more dopamine available at receptor sites in the striatum.

How is L-dopa used in the treatment of Parkinson's disease?

More than two thirds of patients with Parkinson's disease get some significant benefit from the use of L-dopa and in about half of these treatment is dramatically effective. As with most treatments tremor is little affected but the slowing up and rigidity is markedly improved. Unfortunately, L-dopa is one of these drugs where the dose must be very carefully worked out and is different for each patient. The technique is to start with a small dose and increase it every 3–4 days to the highest dose that the patient will tolerate. The major side-effects of L-dopa, in high dosage, include the onset of abnormal movements, nausea and vomiting. Some patients get an uncontrollable twitching involving the facial muscles and tongue. Some patients get a low blood pressure on L-dopa and become dizzy when they stand up. In this case the dosage needs to be reduced.

One recent innovation, which has improved the use of L-dopa, has been the introduction of drugs which prevent it being broken down outside the brain. L-dopa is metabolized by an enzyme called decarboxylase, forming dopamine. This breakdown occurs not only in the brain, where it is part of the essential action of the drug, but also outside the brain in the peripheral tissues. As a result, comparatively little of the dose of L-dopa given to the patient crosses into the brain and gives a therapeutic effect. Drugs have been developed which inhibit the metabolism of L-dopa; these are called decarboxylase inhibitors, e.g. carbidopa. Since these drugs do not themselves enter the brain because of their chemical structure, they very conveniently only inhibit the breakdown of the drug outside the brain, and not inside the brain. Combination tablets of L-dopa with a decarboxylase inhibitor are available and they have certain advantages over using larger doses of L-dopa alone. Patients get less nausea and vomiting and the dyskinesias are also less troublesome.

What about failure to respond to L-dopa?

There are some true failures in whom the Parkinsonism does not respond at all despite adequate dosage. Unfortunately, the natural history of Parkinsonism is to get worse, so that patients who have been on the drug for a while seem to show progressive lack of effect but this is merely the progression of the disease. In the days before L-dopa, stereotaxic surgery of the basal ganglia was sometimes performed to relieve some of the dyskinesia and rigidity. These operations have now been abandoned.

What about drug-induced Parkinsonism?

It is predictable, on pharmacological grounds, that drugs which block dopamine receptors would induce parkinsonism. Indeed it is remarkable that the normal dopaminergic system in the brain can be very substantially blocked by phenothiazine drugs without producing much in the way of parkinsonism. In a way this highlights the quantitative difference between the diseased and the normal dopaminergic system. However, occasionally patients taking antidopaminergic drugs do develop drug-induced parkinsonism. Of course, the primary treatment for this is withdrawal of the drug, but the effect can be dramatically reversed by administration of an anticholinergic drug such as benztropine.

15

Social and addictive drugs

What are social drugs?

Many drugs are not used therapeutically to treat illness, but are taken by individuals for personal satisfaction. Whether such *use* constitutes drug *abuse* is largely one of convention and depends upon a number of factors, the most important of these being:

(1) Whether the individual is harmed by the drug use.

(2) Whether society is harmed by the drug use.

(3) Whether society accepts the drug use as normal or abnormal.

The acceptability of different social drugs in society differs according to time and place. In some countries alcohol is not acceptable, in others cannabis is not acceptable and vice versa. These are largely social judgements and bear little relationship to the pharmacology of the drugs involved.

What is addiction and dependence?

The various definitions of addiction and dependence are imprecise and usually unhelpful. Drug addiction has been dropped as a term and has been replaced by drug dependence, a term favoured by the World Health Organization. *Drug dependence* is defined as a state arising from repeated administration of a drug which results in harm to the individual. Dependence involves three related phenomena, emotional dependence in which there is a desire to take the drug and preoccupation with securing its supply, physical dependence where a withdrawal syndrome occurs if the drug is stopped, and tolerance to the drug where progressively higher doses have to be taken to achieve the same effect.

What drugs produce dependence?

Many common drugs produce dependence, but in some cases this syndrome is a very mild one. For example, most people who regularly drink tea or coffee develop a dependence on caffeine, one of the active ingredients in these beverages. They are usually unaware of this dependence. However, if they are deprived of tea or coffee for 24–48 hours they develop a mild headache which can be relieved by caffeine. According to the strictest definition, therefore, coffee and tea drinkers become dependent upon caffeine. Of course the difference is one of degree because no real harm results from this dependence, as far as we know. On the other extreme there is dependence on opiate narcotic drugs, which can be extreme and sometimes fatal. The commonest social drugs to which dependence is produced are caffeine, alcohol and nicotine, all of which are socially acceptable, and on the other side of the law cannabis or marihuana.

What about tobacco?

More than half the adult population of the Western world smokes tobacco. It is only in the last 40 years or so that the deleterious effect of tobacco smoking on health has been defined. Most dramatically, regular tobacco smokers have a 20-fold higher risk of developing carcinoma of the bronchus than do non-smokers. Furthermore, deaths from other diseases, such as bronchitis and coronary heart disease are also more common in smokers. Smokers have a shorter life expectancy than non-smokers, as a result of these different diseases. The differences are quite large and a smoker is three times more likely to die between the ages of 35 and 65 than is a non-smoker.

What is the pharmacological basis of tobacco smoking?

Although there are many psychological factors involved in tobacco smoking, especially during initiation of the habit when the smoker has to persist in order to eventually enjoy tobacco smoke, there is little doubt that the pharmacological basis of the habit is dependence upon nicotine. Tobacco contains about 2% nicotine which is an alkaloid with potent actions in the body. When tobacco is burned nicotine is transferred to the smoke where it travels in minute droplets of tar. When the smoke is inhaled nicotine is very readily absorbed into the blood after being deposited directly in the lung. Smokers unconsciously adjust their smoking behaviour so as to take in sufficient smoke into their lungs to produce a standard concentration of nicotine in the blood. It appears that the effect of nicotine, which is satisfying to the smoker, is stimulation of acetylcholine receptors within the brain. It seems particularly important that the blood concentration of nicotine should rise and fall rapidly during smoking producing a different stimulation on these receptors second by second. Inhalation of tobacco smoke is a surprising efficient way of getting nicotine from the tobacco leaf into the blood stream. More than 90% of all the nicotine taken into the mouth during smoking is absorbed. Smoking is almost as effective as intravenously injecting nicotine. As the nicotine is absorbed into the lung it bypasses the liver, where oral drugs are metabolized, before exerting a full effect on the brain. Nicotine is a very potent drug, and the amount from one small cigar, if it was extracted and injected intravenously, would be enough to kill an adult man. Most of the nicotine in the cigar curls away from the end of the cigar but up to 10% is absorbed during smoking, over the course of 20–30 minutes. Nevertheless nicotine from tobacco has a rather low 'therapeutic index'.

Most smokers report little change in mood after smoking, and in this the effect is different from other addictive drugs. Tobacco smokers have a feeling of satisfaction which they express either as increased alertness or tranquillity.

What can be done to reduce the harmful effect of smoking?

There is no simple answer to this question and it is a very important one. Basically one has two modes of approach: the first is to reduce consumption of tobacco and the second is to make the tobacco as satisfying but less harmful. As far as reducing consumption is concerned the ideal would be to prevent young people from taking up the habit. Unfortunately cigarette smoking is associated with adult behaviour and is greatly sought after by adolescents as an escape from childhood. Health education has had relatively little impact in this area. Another way of reducing consumption would be to increase the cost of smoking but this has only a temporary effect. The tax on tobacco is already extremely high and the revenue which governments derive from tobacco is so great that this in itself is an obstacle to reducing tobacco consumption. As far as aiding patients to give up smoking after they have been convinced of its deleterious effect, this is extremely difficult. There is a high relapse rate amongst smokers who have given up and permanent 'cure' is rather uncommon. During the acute withdrawal phase nicotine-impregnated chewing gum has shown some success, although the absorption of nicotine from the mouth is much slower than it is from the lung.

The second approach, making cigarettes less toxic, is also problematic. The main toxic material in cigarette smoke is thought to be the tar which contains a number of carcinogenic substances. Tobacco smoke also contains carbon monoxide which is believed to be important in the acceleration of vascular disease seen in smokers. One approach has been to reduce the relative proportion of tar in cigarettes. Unfortunately low tar cigarettes also contain low nicotine, and there is some evidence that smokers smoke more deeply and more of the cigarettes in order to keep their nicotine intake constant. Therefore, this is a self-defeating manoeuvre. Attempts to make artificial tobacco with a low tar content have similarly fallen by the wayside. The logical approach: making a high nicotine, low tar, low carbon monoxide cigarette has not commended itself. In any event it is not certain whether nicotine is without harmful effects. It has recently been suggested that nicotine suppresses prostacyclin formation in blood vessels, and thus might also contribute to vascular disease in smokers.

Are coffee and tea addictive?

In so far as withdrawal of coffee or tea for 24–48 hours produces a withdrawal syndrome consisting of a mild headache, it must be acknowledged that these beverages are dependence producing. It is reassuring to note, however, that no-one has convincingly shown any pathological effects from coffee or tea drinking, and they remain one of the few activities which can be regarded as a harmless pleasure.

SECTION 4

THE AUTONOMIC NERVOUS SYSTEM

16

Drugs and the autonomic nervous system

What is the autonomic nervous system?

The nervous system of the body is traditionally divided into three parts, the central nervous system comprising the brain and spinal cord, the peripheral nervous system including the voluntary, motor and sensory system, and the autonomic system. The latter supplies the internal organs, blood vessels and glands. Both anatomically and pharmacologically the autonomic nervous system is quite different from the peripheral voluntary nervous system. Each autonomic nerve consists of two neurones. The cell body of the first neurone is situated within the central nervous system, and the fibre of this cell runs out to synapse with the second cell, whose axon then terminates on the innervated organ, gland or blood vessel. The neurotransmitters and receptors in this two-cell chain are different from those in the peripheral nervous system.

What is the importance of the autonomic nervous system?

The autonomic nervous system is extremely important because it controls the activity of everything in the body apart from the voluntary muscles. Cardiac rhythm, blood pressure, activity of the kidney and gut, all these things are under autonomic nervous control. Drugs which interfere with the actions of the autonomic nervous system can therefore have very profound effects on physiology. The autonomic nervous system is also important because it was one of the first parts of the nervous system to be investigated systematically by pharmacologists, and a lot more is known about this system than, say, nervous transmission within the central nervous system. In many ways the pharmacology of the autonomic nervous system comprises almost all that was known about drugs before modern synthetic pharmacology really took off 30 years ago. Many of the drugs in common use either affect the sympathetic nervous system or were developed out of drugs which do. A thorough knowledge of the various neurotransmitters, receptors, and drugs acting on the sympathetic nervous system and parasympathetic nervous system gives an excellent grounding in pharmacology.

What is the structure of the autonomic nervous system?

The autonomic nervous system consists of two divisions, and most organs in the body are supplied by nerves from both parts (Figure 6). The first division is called the sympathetic nervous system and the other

The parasympathetic and sympathetic nervous systems

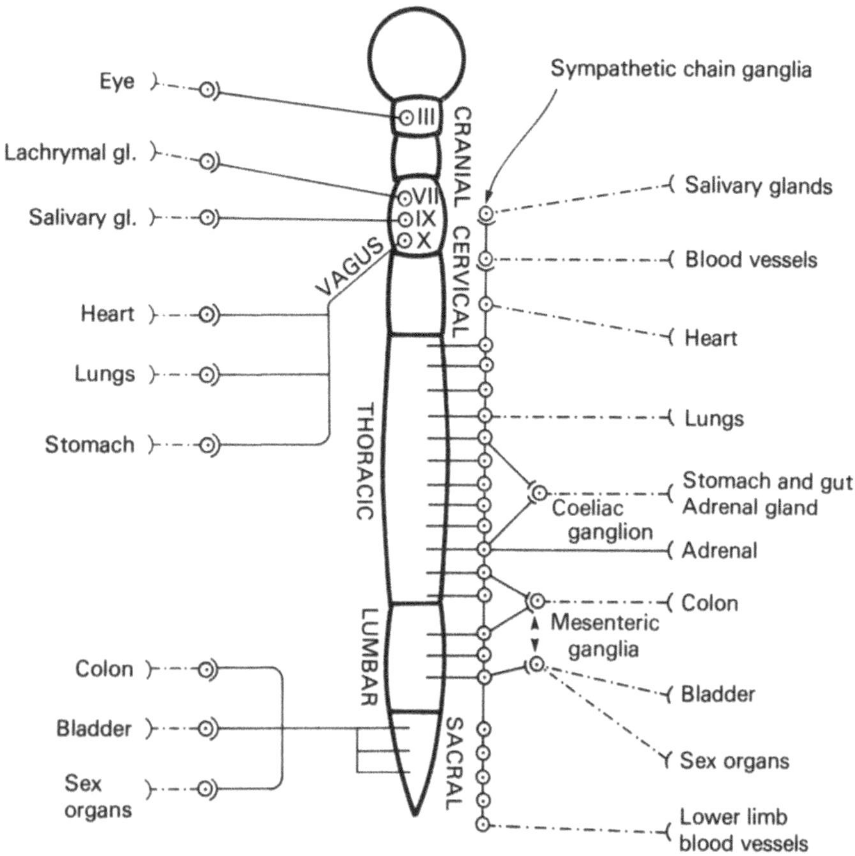

Figure 6 Anatomy of the autonomic nervous system; a diagrammatic representation. Preganglionic neurones bold line, postganglionic neurones interrupted line

part of the system is called the parasympathetic system. In general, stimulation of nerves from both systems have opposite effects on the viscera. For example, stimulating the parasympathetic system to the heart causes slowing of the heart, and stimulating the sympathetic system causes acceleration. Anatomically the two parts of the system are quite distinct. Sympathetic nerves pass out of the spinal cord in the thoracic and lumbar region, passing by the anterior nerve route and then pass to the chain of ganglia lying on either side of the vertebral column. These ganglia consist of nerve cells of the second nerve of the chain. The sympathetic post-ganglionic neurone passes out of the ganglion and then to the organ to be innervated. The parasympathetic system is differently organized, in that the first neurone in the chain is either within the brain or right at the other end of the spinal cord in the sacral cord. In the parasympathetic system, the first neurone has a long axon and the second post-ganglionic neurone is short and is usually situated on the organ to be innervated. The parasympathetic fibres leaving the brain are distributed within four cranial nerves – III, VII, IX and X. The autonomic nervous system also carries sensory fibres to the different organs.

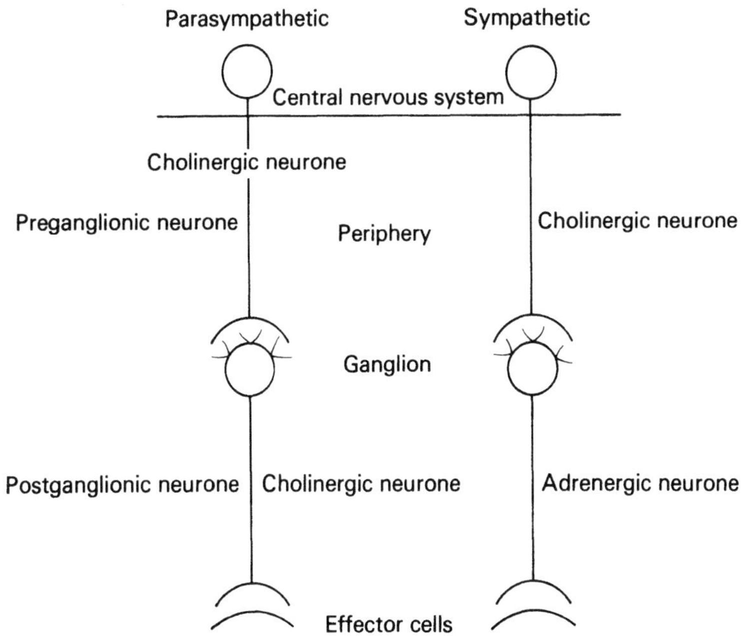

Figure 7 Adrenergic and cholinergic nerves in the parasympathetic and sympathetic systems

What neurotransmitters are there in the parasympathetic system?

Preganglionic neurones of the parasympathetic system liberate acetylcholine at their synapse with the postganglionic neurones. The receptors for acetylcholine at this point are called *nicotinic cholinergic receptors.* The second neurone which terminates on the innervated organ or blood vessel is also cholinergic, in other words it liberates acetylcholine as its neurotransmitter. However, in this case the receptors are of a different type, and although they are stimulated by acetylcholine, they are blocked and stimulated by drugs different from those active at the cholinergic receptors of the ganglion. The post-ganglionic cholinergic receptors are called *muscarinic receptors.* At both cholinergic junctions in the parasympathetic system, the action of acetylcholine is terminated by breakdown catalysed by an enzyme called cholinesterase, which is present in the ganglion and also in the blood (Figure 7).

What drugs act on the parasympathetic system?

A number of different drugs act on the parasympathetic system (Figure 8). Starting at the preganglionic neurone, transmission at the ganglion can be blocked by drugs which competitively antagonize the effect of

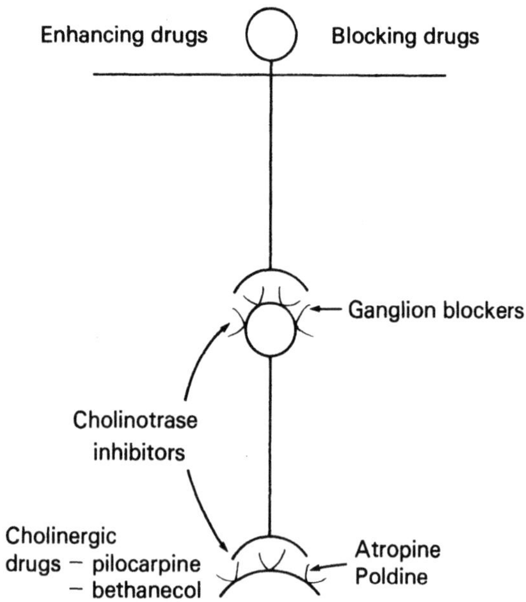

Figure 8 Drugs acting on the parasympathetic system

acetylcholine on nicotinic receptors. These drugs are called ganglion blockers, and such drugs as hexamethonium were originally used for the treatment of high blood pressure. Drugs are also known which block the action of cholinesterase at this junction, either reversibly or irreversibly. The irreversible cholinesterase drugs, the organophosphates are used as insecticides and also as nerve gases. They are intensely poisonous because they enhance transmission at all cholinergic junctions, which include those in the autonomic nervous system, in the voluntary muscles and in the central nervous system. Death occurs from fitting and cessation of respiration.

At the second nerve receptor junction the muscarinic receptors can be blocked by atropine, which is a competitive antagonist at the receptor. Atropine speeds up the heart as it blocks the depressor effect of the vagus on the heart, and dries the mouth as it stops the secretion of saliva. Drugs are also known which simulate the effect of acetylcholine at muscarinic receptors, such as pilocarpine, bethanechol and propantheline. These drugs are used in the treatment of glaucoma and as antispasmodics in the gut.

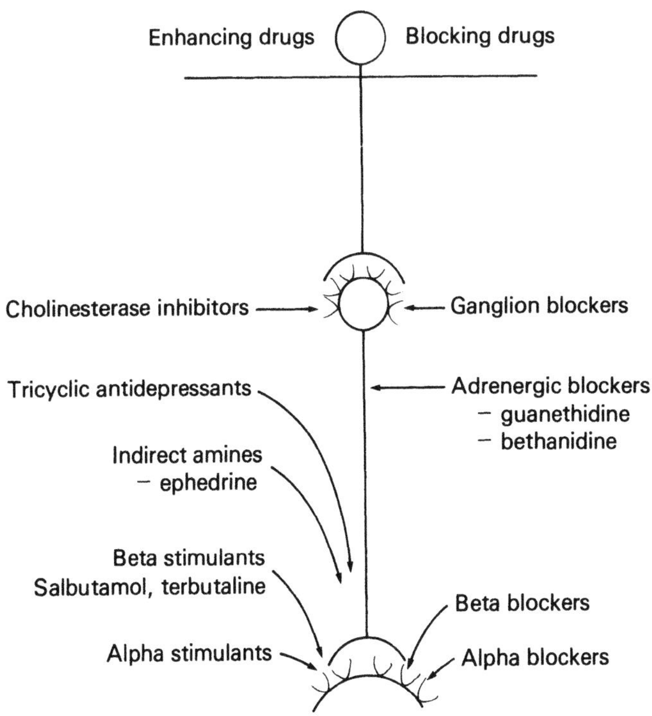

Figure 9 Drugs acting on the sympathetic system

What neurotransmitters are there in the sympathetic nervous system?

The sympathetic system has a similar pharmacology to the parasympathetic system, so far as the first neurone or preganglionic neurone is concerned (Figure 9). Transmission at the sympathetic ganglion is exactly the same as at the parasympathetic ganglia, acetylcholine being liberated onto nicotinic receptors. However, the postganglionic neurone in the sympathetic system is totally different and liberates noradrenaline. There is one specialized gland innervated by the sympathetic system and this is the adrenal gland, where stimulation of the preganglionic neurone leads to release of not only noradrenaline but of adrenaline. The medulla of the adrenal gland liberates these two powerful drugs into the blood stream, and they produce widespread effects, particularly on the cardiovascular system, when the adrenal medulla is stimulated.

What receptors are there for noradrenaline and adrenaline

The noradrenaline liberated from the postganglionic sympathetic neurone acts on its effector cell by stimulating receptors. There are at least two different types of receptor for noradrenaline, so-called α- and β-receptors. Drugs are known which will act selectively on either one of these receptors and both are useful in medical practice. Stimulation of α-receptors by noradrenaline produces constriction of blood vessels and hence a rise in blood pressure. Stimulation of β-receptors causes relaxation of the bronchi and blood vessels, and an increase in the heart rate. Some of the tissues innervated by the sympathetic system have a preponderance of α-receptors and some a preponderance of β-receptors. It is also known that the β-receptors differ slightly in different tissues. Hence on the heart the beta receptors are β_1 type, whereas on the bronchi there are β-receptors, and drugs are known which will selectively block responses at either type of receptor. All these drugs have particular uses because of their selectivity.

What are the pharmacological actions of adrenaline?

Adrenaline causes acceleration of the heart, which may be perceived as palpitation, a rise in blood pressure and the relaxation of the bronchial tree. All of these events occur when adrenaline is naturally liberated from the adrenal gland, which occurs during excitement or shock. Liberation of adrenaline is the cause of pounding of the heart during excitement or danger. Acceleration of the heart is caused by the adrenaline combining with the β-receptors on the heart. In therapeutics, adrenaline is used as an injection for the acute treatment of anaphylactic shock or bronchial asthma. For this purpose adrenaline is injected intramuscularly. It is important that the drug is not given into a vein because large doses of adrenaline given in this way can stimulate the heart so much as to cause an arrhythmia. Adrenaline can be given by direct intracardiac puncture in cardiac arrest when asystole is present.

What is the pharmacology of noradrenaline?

Noradrenaline is the natural neurotransmitter released from post-ganglionic sympathetic neurones. Hence intravenous injection of the drug mimics the effect of stimulating the entire sympathetic nervous system. The most important action is to increase the blood pressure. It does this by stimulating α-receptors on blood vessels. Noradrenaline is not used in therapeutics.

What other drugs have direct actions on α-and β-receptors?

Drugs which stimulate α-receptors are known experimentally, but they do not have any value in therapeutics. However, drugs which stimulate β-receptors are useful because they can be used as bronchodilators in patients with asthma. Since both the lung and the heart possess β-receptors, there has been a search for drugs which will stimulate lung β-receptors producing bronchodilatation, and yet have little effect on cardiac β-receptors where they will cause arrhythmias and acceleration of the heart. It has been found that the β-receptors in the heart and lung are structurally different, so that it is possible to produce drugs which are selective on one or the other receptor. The β-receptor in the lung is called a β_2-receptor and drugs selective for this β-receptor include salbutamol and terbutaline. These are synthetic drugs which are known as β_2-agonists. They have largely replaced isoprenaline, another synthetic drug which stimulates both β_1- and β_2-receptors. Salbutamol and terbutaline can be given by mouth, and also by inhaler where they directly stimulate the bronchi. Unfortunately, there are also β-receptors on voluntary muscle and when given in large doses, these β-stimulant drugs for asthma also cause tremor.

What about β-blocking drugs?

There is now a large number of drugs which block the effect of adrenaline or noradrenaline on β-receptors. These drugs were originally developed to reduce the effect of sympathetic stimulation on the heart, reduce cardiac work and hence be effective in treating angina pectoris where the heart has a reduced blood supply due to disease of the coronary arteries. β-Blockers are effective treatments of angina pectoris but they have also been found to be useful in a number of other diseases, and in particular in high blood pressure. The first β-blocker, to be used successfully, was propranolol but there are now a variety of other β-blockers with slightly different properties. Propranolol blocks both β_1- and β_2-receptors. Blocking β_2-receptors in the lung does not cause any disability in normal individuals, but in patients with asthma it can cause bronchoconstriction. Therefore a search was made for drugs which would selectively block the β_1-receptors in the heart and not the β_2-receptors in the lung. This search has been successful, and there are now a number of drugs, such as atenolol or metoprolol which are relatively selective for the cardiac receptors. However, in severe asthmatics they still produce some degree of bronchoconstriction. β-Blockers are very useful and widely used drugs in medicine. They reduce arterial pressure, slow the heart and have some metabolic effects, which appear to be of little consequence.

What are the side-effects of β-blockers?

The side-effects of the β-blockers, apart from precipitation of asthma, include worsening of heart failure. Patients with heart failure often have an increased sympathetic drive which is in fact stimulating the heart to as great an effort as is possible to make. When β-blockers are introduced this drive is withdrawn and the heart failure may get worse. Another common side-effect of β-blockers is the production of cold hands and feet. This is an effect of peripheral vasoconstriction and reduced cardiac output. It can be troublesome but many patients choose to tolerate the effect rather than stop the drug.

17

Antihypertensives

What is hypertension?

Hypertension or high blood pressure is a condition in which the patient is at risk of developing heart disease, kidney failure and stroke as a result of persistently high blood pressure. It must be remembered that there is a tremendous difference between a high blood pressure and having high blood pressure. Even in perfectly normal individuals occasional high blood pressure readings are seen during stress or exercise. However, in patients with the condition of high blood pressure, the pressure is consistently and persistently elevated.

What are the consequences of hypertension?

High blood pressure can precipitate a variety of problems in the heart, kidney and circulation. The higher the blood pressure the shorter the life expectancy (Figure 10). Stroke is six times more common in patients with hypertension, and heart attack about three times more common. Patients with very high blood pressure tend to die from malignant hypertension or from progressive kidney failure. In general, hypertension does not cause symptoms although it is traditionally associated with headache, dizziness, tenseness and anxiety.

Are there different types of hypertension?

There are many different ways of classifying hypertensive patients. In most patients no cause can be found for the raised pressure, but in a minority of patients the blood pressure is raised due to some underlying problem such as kidney disease. There are also endocrine causes for hypertension. Perhaps the most useful way of classifying patients is according to the severity of the illness, and whether damage has already occurred to the so-called target organs, brain, heart and kidneys, because of a persistently raised blood pressure. There is one very severe form of hypertension called malignant hypertension, where small blood vessels of the body suddenly become unable to take the strain of increased pressure and start to break up. This causes death within a few months, and the condition can be diagnosed by examining the arterioles of the retina with an ophthalmoscope. Here the small blood vessels of the body can be seen directly, and failure of these vessels to contain the pressure is evident. Malignant hypertension is a crisis situation which must be treated very vigorously if the patient is not to succumb.

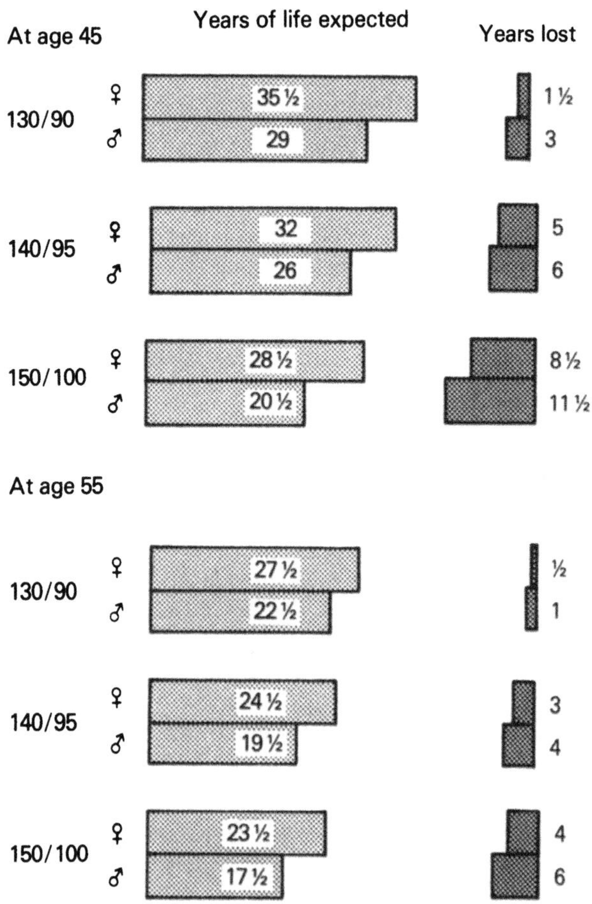

Figure 10 Reduction in life expectancy associated with mildly raised blood pressure, which remains untreated. Data courtesy of 'The Metropolitan Life Assurance Company', New York

What factors normally regulate blood pressure?

The level of the patient's blood pressure is a balance between the output of the heart and the tone in the peripheral blood vessels through which the blood flows, the so-called peripheral resistance. Blood pressure is maintained, within narrow limits, in normal individuals by a large number of different regulatory systems, mostly dependent upon control by the autonomic nervous system. Adrenergic nerves to the resistance vessels control their tone and the innervation of the heart controls its output. The kidney is also important in the regulation of blood pressure, first because it regulates the amount of salt and water removed from the body and hence the volume of blood in the circulation, and secondly, because it produces at least one hormone, renin, which acts to control the tone of the peripheral blood vessels. In most patients with hypertension no specific fault can be found in any of these mechanisms, and it is probable that the blood pressure is just set too high as a result of genetic mechanisms.

How is hypertension treated?

Prior to the early 1950s there was no effective treatment for hypertension, but since then there has been a tremendous advance in pharmacology, and now very many drugs are available which effectively lower blood pressure and are used for treating hypertension. Nowadays the treatment of hypertension is almost exclusively with drugs. Surgical treatment of patients with hypertension is restricted to those who have some endocrine tumour responsible for causing the high blood pressure, such as phaeochromocytoma or Cushing's tumour of the adrenal. Occasionally when renal disease is responsible for the hypertension, this can be ameliorated by surgery, but for the majority of patients hypertension is treated with drugs and since the condition is a chronic one, these drugs have to be continued for the whole of the patient's life.

When is it desirable to treat high blood pressure?

In general, the higher the blood pressure the greater the risk of the consequences of hypertension. Thus there is no argument that patients with very high blood pressure should be treated and patients with malignant hypertension should be treated immediately as an emergency. However, there is a large number of patients who have only a mildly raised blood pressure and in consequence only have a slightly increased risk of complications such as stroke or heart attack. It is likely that treating these patients would also benefit them, but the inconvenience and cost has to be balanced against the small benefits that they would receive. At the moment there is some argument about how severe high blood pressure has to be before it should be treated. In general, patients with a diastolic blood pressure of 105 mmHg or more are almost always treated. Some doctors treat patients whose diastolic pressure is consistently 95 mmHg or above. In elderly patients there is less to be gained by treating hypertension, and side-effects tend to be more prominent. Most doctors only treat elderly patients if the hypertension is causing some immediate problem, such as heart failure.

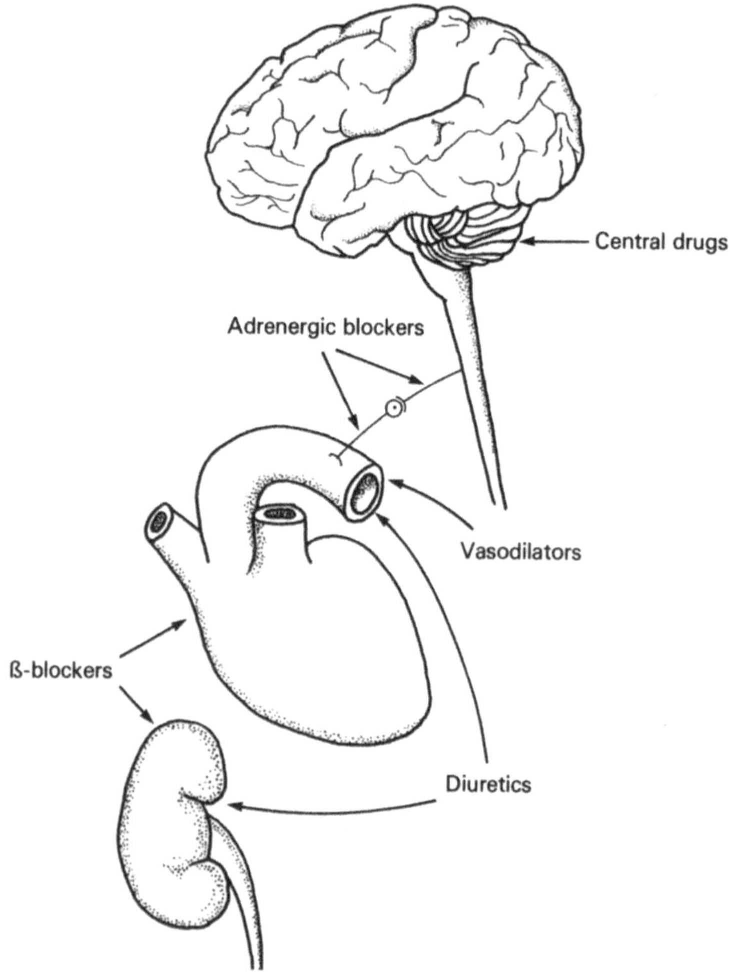

Figure 11 Site of action of five main types of antihypertensive drugs

What drugs are available for treating hypertension?

Historically the first drugs which were used for treating hypertension were the ganglion blockers. These drugs interfere with the activity of the whole autonomic nervous system, the parasympathetic and the sympathetic system. As a result, they cause many side-effects and they have been replaced by other more specific drugs which interfere more specifically with the sympathetic nervous system. The next drugs to be developed were adrenergic neurone blocking drugs such as guanethidine or bethanidine. These drugs interfere with transmission in the postganglionic sympathetic neurone, and hence relieve sympathetic vasoconstriction of the peripheral arterioles. They have one major side-effect and that is that they cause postural hypotension. That is the blood pressure is lower when the patient stands up than when he or she is lying down. This occurs simply because the sympathetic nervous system is activated when the patient stands up more than when the patient lies down. The consequence of this postural hypotension is that patients become faint and dizzy on standing up and this is a major problem. Therefore, these drugs have also been phased out. The modern therapy of hypertension is largely based on three different types of drugs (Figure 11), firstly the diuretics, secondly β-blocking drugs and thirdly vasodilators. In reserve are a number of drugs which act within the brain to diminish the activity of the sympathetic nervous system, the so-called centrally acting drugs.

What drugs are used in mild hypertension?

Mild hypertension is usually treated either with a diuretic or with a β-blocker (discussed in Chapter 16). These drugs block the action of noradrenaline released from adrenergic neurones at β-receptors on the heart, bronchi and blood vessels. In hypertension, their action is thought to be in reducing the cardiac output by slowing the heart and reducing its force of contraction. In practice, β-blockers are very effective drugs in hypertension and are well tolerated by patients with few side-effects. β-Blockers have a long duration of action and can be given once a day, often as a single tablet. Their main disadvantage is that they cannot be given to patients with asthma. In addition β-blockers sometimes induce heart failure, and if the patient has intermittent claudication, they may make this worse.

What β-blockers are used?

The tendency now is to use β-blockers which are β_1-receptor selective. These drugs have more effect on the heart than on the bronchi. Such drugs include atenolol and metoprolol but non-selective drugs affecting both β_1- and β_2-receptors, such as propranolol and oxprenolol, are still widely used.

What are the advantages and disadvantages of diuretics?

Diuretics have been used for the treatment of hypertension for about 20 years, although it is still not entirely clear how they work to lower the blood pressure. Although their most investigated site of action is in the kidney, where they cause an increase in salt and water excretion, they also relax the blood vessels somewhat and this is probably the way they act in hypertension. Diuretics have a large advantage in that they cause very few side-effects for the patient to complain of, apart from having to pass urine soon after taking the tablets. However, taken over a period of years, diuretics cause a number of metabolic side-effects which can be troublesome. These include a form of diabetes, gout due to impaired excretion of uric acid by the kidney and a low serum potassium. A low serum potassium is of no particular importance in itself, but it does predispose the patient to toxicity if he or she is taking digoxin in addition. Because of these metabolic side-effects, many clinicians prefer to start treatment with a β-blocker, especially as there is some suggestive evidence that β-blockers may reduce the incidence of myocardial infarction.

What about more severe hypertension?

Most patients with moderate or severe hypertension cannot have their blood pressure reduced to normal while taking a single drug. Combination therapy with several different drugs is usual in these patients. The first combination used is to add a diuretic to a β-blocker. If the patient's blood pressure is still not well controlled, the usual drug added next is a vasodilator such as hydralazine or prazosin which reduce vascular tone in the peripheral resistance vessels. They are not used on their own in hypertension because they provoke a reflex acceleration of the heart. This is not a problem when the patient is taking a β-blocker. Hydralazine is a drug which should not be used in doses higher than 200 mg/day because it can provoke a syndrome known as drug-induced lupus erythematosus. This resembles the collagen disease but is reversible when the drug is stopped.

What about other drugs for use in hypertension?

Other useful drugs in hypertension include the centrally acting drugs such as methyldopa or clonidine. These drugs act by reducing the sympathetic nervous activity by an action within the brain at central circuits. They are very active drugs and do not cause as much postural hypotension as the adrenergic blocking drugs. However, they have different side-effects, particularly sedation and a dry mouth. Some patients tolerate these effects reasonably well, others find them very unpleasant. One particular problem of clonidine is that if it is stopped abruptly the patient gets a rebound hypertension with tremendous sympathetic discharge, raised blood pressure and cardiac acceleration. As with all the antihypertensive drugs, patients taking them must understand their treatment, comply with the proper doses of drugs and continue to take them regularly.

What is malignant hypertension and how is it treated?

Malignant hypertension is a medical emergency, where there is evidence that the small blood vessels of the body are breaking up under the strain of the high blood pressure. The vision is particularly affected, and small blood vessels at the back of the eye can be seen to be leaking blood and serum. In the brain, similar changes occur and the patient may go into coma. There is often a rapid deterioration in renal function. When the diagnosis of malignant hypertension is made, the blood pressure must be lowered as a matter of urgency. In the past, patients were treated with intravenous drugs, and the blood pressure reduced with vasodilators such as diazoxide or sodium nitroprusside or ganglion-blocking drugs, such as pentolinium. These very effectively lowered the blood pressure, but in some cases the abrupt fall in pressure precipitated a stroke. Therefore, it is now more usual to use large oral doses of drugs, and to reduce the pressure over 2–3 days, allowing the vascular system time to adjust to the new lower pressure.

18

Cardiac drugs

How are drugs used in heart disease?

Drugs are used in three situations, to treat heart failure, to treat the irregularity of the heart rhythm and to treat cardiac ischaemia.

What is heart failure?

Heart failure occurs when the cardiac output fails to perfuse the organs of the body with an adequate blood supply. In heart failure a patient becomes breathless because of oedema and congestion of the lungs. The kidneys are poorly perfused, and as a result retain salt and water leading to oedema, particularly of the ankles. As the cardiac output falls, engorgement of the liver occurs and blood can be seen accumulating in the veins of the neck. In heart failure the patient becomes breathless on the slightest exertion.

What drugs are used to treat heart failure?

There are three different approaches to treating heart failure. The first is to increase the output of the heart by giving a drug which increases cardiac contraction. These drugs are known as *inotropic agents.* The second approach is to use a diuretic which increases the output of salt and water by the kidney. The third approach is to lower the peripheral resistance in the circulation and reduce the amount of work that the heart has to do in perfusing the tissues. Vasodilators are used for this purpose.

What inotropic agents are there?

There are only two types of inotropic agents, digitalis-type drugs and the more recently discovered catecholamine-like drugs dopamine and dobutamine. These latter agents have to be given intravenously, and work by stimulating those β-receptors on the heart particularly concerned with cardiac contraction. They have some use in acute heart failure such as that following cardiac surgery. However, in the more common form of chronic heart failure digitalis is still the drug of choice.

What is digitalis and how does it work?

Digitalis is a cardiac glycoside which has been used in the treatment of heart failure for almost 200 years. It is a natural product obtained from the foxglove. Nowadays, one particular digitalis glycoside, digoxin, is used. The effect of digoxin is only seen on a heart which shows failure, and it does not have any effect on the normal heart. In the failing heart digoxin increases the force of contraction of the heart, slows the heart down, probably by an action on the vagus nerve, and also depresses the conduction of the cardiac impulse across the atrioventricular node. This slowing of the heart is an important action in patients with atrial fibrillation. Digoxin binds to the heart muscle to produce this effect and accumulation of the drug occurs. The dosage of digoxin has to be carefully adjusted as it is a drug with a rather low therapeutic index.

What are the toxic effects of digitalis?

In a patient who is receiving too much digitalis nausea and vomiting is a prominent feature. Bradycardia, when a heart rate drops below 60, can occur due to the excessive effect of the drug on the bundle of His. If the pulse rate is below 60 digitalis should not be given. Occasionally digitalis causes ventricular extrasystoles, and in a patient with sinus rhythm these can be detected as coupled beats. This effect is thought to be due to digitalis increasing the excitability of the ventricles. Again they are an indication to stop the drug temporarily. With prolonged overdosage patients may complain of yellow vision, an effect on the retina. Digitalis toxicity on the heart is exacerbated by low serum potassium, a common side-effect of diuretics which are usually given with digoxin. Patients on digoxin should therefore be given adequate potassium supplements, such as Slow-K.

What is digitalization?

It is usual when starting digitalis to give a large initial dose followed by a smaller dose, until the patient shows a satisfactory response. A typical regime would be to give 0.5 mg digoxin stat followed by 0.25 mg three times a day for 2–3 days. The maintenance dose in most patients is around 0.25 mg daily. Patients who have impaired renal function require smaller doses, as do elderly patients, because digoxin is excreted by the kidney and accumulation occurs in renal failure. For rapid digitalization intravenous preparations are available but they are almost never needed.

What other digitalis glycosides are there?

There are several different glycosides of digitalis, apart from digoxin. Digitoxin is very similar to digoxin but has a longer halflife and it is therefore more difficult to adjust the dose. There are several glycosides such as strophanthus and ouabain which can be given intravenously. They are rarely used.

How are diuretics and vasodilators used in cardiac failure?

In mild cardiac failure a diuretic may be all that is necessary. Administration of diuretics reduces body weight in patients with cardiac failure and may totally abolish dependent oedema. A thiazide diuretic can be given orally and is the first-line drug. In patients with resistant oedema, a loop diuretic with a more powerful action, such as frusemide, is commonly used, and in patients with chronic resistant oedema spironolactone can be introduced.

Use of vasodilators in patients with heart failure is still somewhat experimental. Rapidly acting vasodilators such as prazosin and hydralazine are sometimes effective in treating acute heart failure.

What about left ventricular failure?

Left ventricular failure, or pulmonary oedema, is a dramatic event where a patient becomes suddenly extremely breathless and froths at the mouth. The patient becomes acutely distressed, is unable to breathe, and if the attack cannot be treated effectively this may be a fatal event. It is a medical emergency, and once seen left ventricular failure is never forgotten. What happens is that the failing left ventricle allows blood to back up in the lung and the increased venous pressure in the lung allows transudation of fluid into the lung. The patient cannot breathe because of the fluid, which may froth up the trachea and out of the mouth. Acute left ventricular failure occurs in heart disease and a variety of other conditions, and especially after a massive myocardial infarction. Treatment of left ventricular failure is with intravenous injection of frusemide, which is often dramatically effective. Another very useful drug is aminophylline, which is also given intravenously in this situation. Aminophylline works by reducing the peripheral resistance and improving the left ventricular output. The dose is 200–400 mg over 5–10 minutes intravenously. In patients who get repeated attacks of left ventricular failure at night, aminophylline can be given as a suppository last thing at night.

What is a cardiac arrhythmia?

The normal rhythm of the heart is sinus rhythm. In sinus rhythm the contractile stimulus starts at the pacemaker in the sinoatrial node. The impulse to contract then passes over both atria through the atrioventricular node, down the bundle of His and into the muscles of both ventricles. Hence the atria contract before the ventricles. This orderly sequence of events can be disturbed and there are many different disorders of rhythm known as cardiac arrhythmias.

What cardiac arrhythmias are there?

There are several different classifications. The simplest way of classifying them is into those that cause fast heart rates and those that cause slow heart rates. The causes of bradycardia (slow heart rate) include drug treatment with digitalis and β-blockers, sinus bradycardia in young athletic people and heart block. In heart block there is a disturbance of the atrioventricular node so that not all atrial contractions are followed by a ventricular contraction.

There are many more causes of fast heart rate arrhythmias. In some the defect is in the atria, the so-called supraventricular arrhythmias, and in others the defect is in the ventricles, ventricular tachycardias. In the supraventricular arrhythmias an irritable part of the atria fires at a higher rate than the sinus node, producing three different types of arrhythmia, atrial fibrillation, the most common where the heart rate is irregularly irregular, atrial flutter and atrial tachycardia which is usually paroxysmal. Ventricular tachycardia is more dangerous than any of these conditions because it can lead to ventricular fibrillation where the cardiac output effectively ceases.

What drugs are used to treat arrhythmias?

Bradycardia due to heart block was formerly treated with β-stimulant drugs, which increase the ventricular rate. However, heart block is now almost always treated with a pacemaker, and the isoprenaline preparations once commonly used are now obsolete. Treatment of the tachycardias is much more complex. Digitalis is the drug of choice in atrial fibrillation, atrial flutter and paroxysmal atrial tachycardia. However digitalis should not be given to patients with ventricular arrhythmias as it can make them worse.

What other drugs are used in cardiac arrhythmias?

(1) Local anaesthetic drugs. These drugs such as lignocaine and mexiletine suppress cardiac excitability. Lignocaine is particularly valuable in suppressing ventricular excitability following myocardial infarction, and must be given intravenously. In overdosage, lignocaine has toxic central effects and can provoke fits. Mexiletine is similar to lignocaine and can be given orally.

(2) Quinidine-like drugs. Quinidine and procainamide also reduce overexcitability of cardiac muscle and are valuable in ventricular arrhythmias. Both can be given orally.

(3) β-Blockers. Blocking cardiac β-receptors reduces cardiac excitability, and β-blockers can also be used to treat paroxysmal atrial tachycardias as well as ventricular arrhythmias.

What drugs are used for coronary heart disease?

Coronary heart disease is extremely common, and in the majority of patients there is no effective way of preventing its onset or progression. The underlying cause of the disease still remains unknown, although a great deal of research is being undertaken. Drugs are useful, however, in managing some of the complications of coronary heart disease, namely angina of effort and myocardial infarction.

What is angina of effort?

Angina is a characteristic pain, usually a crushing pain in the chest radiating to the jaw or arm, which is brought on by effort and is due to ischaemia of the heart. Occasionally, similar pain occurs when the patient is not exerting himself and here the heart ischaemia is thought to be due not to increased oxygen demand by the heart but by the coronary artery itself going into spasm. This latter type of angina is called 'variant angina'.

What drugs are used for the treatment of angina?

Nitrites, β-blockers and calcium antagonists are all used. The first-line drug in angina is a nitrite; these are drugs which act on smooth muscle causing it to relax. There are a number of different nitrite drugs all having a similar pharmacology but some having a prolonged effect. The most commonly used drug is glyceryl trinitrate. It is the same substance as the explosive TNT. In medicine very small amounts of the active drug are absorbed onto a chalky base and used as tablets. Glyceryl trinitrate is taken by mouth and is absorbed from the mucous membranes under the tongue. Given in this way, the drug is very rapidly absorbed and causes a generalized fall in blood pressure which rapidly relieves anginal pain. The drug may also cause some relaxation of the coronary artery. Other nitrites such as sorbide nitrate and pentaerythritol tetranitrate can be taken orally. In general, if the chest pain on exertion does not respond to sucking a glyceryl trinitrate tablet, there is probably some error in the diagnosis. A common difficulty with glyceryl trinitrate is that the patient may get a throbbing headache after its use and it may be necessary for the dose to be reduced.

When are β-blockers used in angina?

β-Blockers reduce cardiac work and hence cardiac oxygen demand. In this way they can prevent the onset of angina and β-blockers are very effective at this. A small dose is given to start with, and care is exercised so that the patient does not develop heart failure. If β-blockers are given regularly to angina patients and if patients on them do still develop anginal attacks, then these can be treated at the time with glyceryl trinitrate.

What other drugs can be used?

Recently calcium antagonist drugs have been developed for use in angina. Nifedipine is such a drug. The drugs work by antagonizing the influx of calcium into cardiac muscle which occurs after the muscle is excited. Nifedipine reduces the force and velocity of cardiac contraction and thus reduces cardiac oxygen demand. It also relaxes smooth muscle elsewhere in the body, and slightly lowers the blood pressure. Nifedipine is said to be particularly effective in variant angina where spasm of the coronary artery is thought to be important. However, it causes flushing, dizziness and headaches and may produce cardiac failure as a result of in reducing cardiac contraction.

What about the treatment of acute myocardial infarction?

Patients with acute myocardial infarction are in pain and apprehensive. A major cause of death in acute myocardial infarction is a cardiac arrhythmia leading to cardiac arrest. The next commonest cause of death is intractable cardiac failure. Both of these complications are most readily treated in a cardiac care unit, where the heart rhythm can be monitored and appropriate antiarrhythmic drugs given if an arrhythmia occurs. Pain relief should be prompt and effective using an opiate analgesic. Other treatment given to patients with acute coronary thrombosis depend on the clinical circumstance. Anticoagulant drugs are no longer used as they have been shown to be ineffective.

19

Drugs for asthma

What is asthma?

Asthma is a disease where attacks of wheezing occur which can seriously interfere with breathing. The wheeze is due to a narrowing of the bronchi, caused by spasm of bronchial muscle and blockage of the bronchi by mucous plugs and inflammatory fluid.

How is asthma treated?

Drugs are important in asthma, but general measures such as avoiding allergens and precipitating psychological factors are also relevant. There are four different types of drugs which can be used: bronchodilators, steroids, mucolytics and cromoglycate.

What drugs are useful as bronchodilators?

There are three main types of drug which act as bronchodilators. They are all thought to act by relaxing bronchial smooth muscle. The drugs can be classified as:

(1) β-Adrenoceptor agonist drugs, such as salbutamol.
(2) Theophylline and related drugs.
(3) Atropine-like drugs.

What β-mimetic drugs are used as bronchodilators?

Ephedrine is a drug which has been used in asthma for 4000 years, and was known to the ancient Chinese as the herb *ma haung*. It acts orally and is now known to act by releasing noradrenaline from sympathetic nerve endings. However, ephedrine has central effects, causing stimulation and apprehension. The modern equivalents of ephedrine are adrenaline-like drugs which have been refined to have selected actions on the bronchial β_2-adrenoceptors, rather than the cardiac β_1-receptors which speed the heart. Such drugs include salbutamol, terbutaline and isoetharine. These drugs are active by mouth but are best given by aerosol inhaler. This maximizes the drug delivered directly to the bronchi, while minimizing such systemic side-effects as cardiac acceleration and tremor of the voluntary muscles. Selective drugs have virtually displaced the non-selective β-mimetic drugs such as isoprenaline and orciprenaline.

How does theophylline work?

Theophylline is a plant alkaloid which relaxes smooth muscle other than that in blood vessels, and decreases airway resistance especially in asthma. The drug is believed to act by inhibiting the enzyme phosphodiesterase, and hence the breakdown of cyclic AMP, an important intracellular messenger. Stimulation of β-receptors increases cellular cyclic AMP so the action of β-stimulants and theophylline are additive. In asthma theophylline can be given intravenously, in the form of aminophylline (an ethylene diamine salt of theophylline) or as various salts such as choline theophyllinate, which are active orally and are formulated to reduce gastric irritation of the native drug.

What atropine-like drugs can be used as bronchodilators?

Anticholinergics block the vagal stimulation to bronchial muscle and decrease bronchial secretion. Unfortunately this often makes the bronchosecretion more tenacious. Recently, an inhaler containing the anticholinergic drug ipratropium has been introduced.

When are steroids used in asthma?

Steroids are very effective in asthma but they are used as little as possible. Once a patient is commenced on oral treatment with steroids it is very difficult to stop the drug, and the side-effects of the steroids, such as moon face, hairiness, fragile bones, hypertension and diabetes, are extremely severe. Steroids are therefore reserved for status asthmaticus and very severe asthmatics who are unresponsive to other drugs. Recently it has been shown that steroids can be given safely in small doses via a bronchial inhaler. Used in this way the local steroid does not result in the usual systemic side-effects; but unfortunately the inhaler is not quite as effective as the oral drug.

What is cromoglycate?

Cromoglycate is not a bronchodilator, but prevents some allergic and inflammatory responses. It is believed to act by inhibiting the release of histamine and other asthmagenic substances from mast cells. Cromoglycate is not absorbed from the gut and has to be inhaled directly as a powder into the lungs using a 'spin' inhaler.

What about mucolytics?

Mucolytics such as bromhexine are drugs which increase broncho-secretion and make it less tenacious. Their main use is in bronchitis but they can be useful in asthma.

What is status asthmaticus?

Status asthmaticus is a serious medical emergency where the patient has such severe bronchospasm that respiratory failure is possible, particularly when the patient begins to be exhausted by the efforts of breathing. The usual way of managing this emergency is to administer humidified oxygen and full intravenous doses of β-stimulant drugs. Other drugs given include intravenous aminophylline and steroids. Unfortunately steroids take at least 8 hours to have any action in asthma, so oral prednisolone is just as effective as intravenously injected hydrocortisone.

Can asthma be fatal?

There is an old adage that 'no-one ever dies of asthma'. Certainly patients can be extremely ill with status asthmaticus for days on end and still recover completely. However, asthma must be treated seriously and is certainly a distressing condition for the patients. In the 1960s there was an epidemic of sudden death amongst young asthmatics which was eventually shown to be due to excessive use of high dosage isoprenaline aerosols; this caused death by producing cardiac arrhythmias. Selective β_2-agonist drugs now used in inhalers are somewhat safer, but patients should be warned not to exceed the stated dose, even if the bronchospasm is not relieved.

SECTION 5

HORMONES AND PREGNANCY

20

The endocrine system

What is meant by the endocrine system?

The endocrine system comprises those glands whose function is to liberate hormones into the blood. Hormones are chemicals which act as internal messengers in the body, their function being to regulate activity in tissues distant to the glands secreting them. The endocrine system is essentially an information system. As discussed in the section on the central nervous system, cells in the body can only communicate with one another by releasing chemical messengers. In the nervous system the distance the chemical or neurotransmitter traverses is minute and the time for the message to be transmitted is extremely short. In the endocrine system the chemical transmitter or hormone may travel right across the body to its target cell, and the transmission time may be very prolonged. In general then, the nervous system conveys rapidly changing information and the endocrine system is responsible for slowly changing information.

How does drug treatment affect the endocrine system?

The endocrine system is an important target for therapy. In the first place many important functions are directly controlled by hormonal secretion. Metabolic rate, growth, sexual activity, appetite are all hormonally regulated. Drugs can be devised which work on hormones or their receptors. In the second place, the endocrine system often malfunctions and requires manipulation. Failure of endocrine glands to produce sufficient hormone can be treated very precisely, by replacement with synthetic hormones or hormones extracted from human or animal tissue. Overactivity of an endocrine gland may be treated in some cases by drugs which reduce hormonal secretion by the gland or drugs which antagonize the released hormone.

What endocrine glands are there?

It is a useful oversimplification to regard the various endocrine glands as belonging to three main groups. The first group comprises the pituitary and three other glands which are controlled by it, namely the gonads, the thyroid and the adrenal cortex. The next group comprises the large endocrine glands, which are not controlled by the pituitary. These comprise the adrenal medulla, the pancreas and the parathyroids. Finally there are organs which are endocrine glands in addition to their other predominant function. Many organs produce circulating hormones in addition to their apparent primary function. An example of this would be the kidney which produces renin and erythropoietin, the lung which produces prostacyclin and the alimentary canal which produces a whole host of peptide hormones which control digestion.

What hormones does the pituitary produce?

The pituitary comprises two quite separate glands. The posterior pituitary is a neural structure which produces oxytocin and vasopressin, otherwise known as antidiuretic hormone (ADH). The anterior pituitary is 'the conductor of the endocrine orchestra' and produces six hormones, growth hormone (GH), prolactin, adrenocorticotrophin (ACTH), thyrotropin (TSH) and two gonadotrophins, luteinizing hormone (LH) and follicle-stimulating hormone (FSH). Through these hormones the anterior pituitary gland regulates the function of three other endocrine glands, namely the gonads, the thyroid and the adrenal cortex.

What does ACTH do?

ACTH is a protein produced by the anterior pituitary which stimulates the adrenal cortex to produce corticosteroids. The adrenal/pituitary system works by *feedback inhibition*. This means that the pituitary senses the level of corticosteroids in blood and increases ACTH production if the level falls. Conversely if a patient is given corticosteroids therapeutically, then this suppresses ACTH release. Because of this regulating system, long term treatment with steroids is hazardous to the patient if it is stopped abruptly. In this case, the suppressed pituitary may not respond rapidly enough to provoke the adrenal to start producing steroids again.

At one time ACTH was used as a drug in preference to oral corticosteroids such as prednisolone. It was thought that ACTH was more physiological in that it stimulated the body to secrete natural adrenal steroids. However, ACTH has to be injected and there is no good evidence of any greater efficacy or lesser side-effects when ACTH is used rather than oral steroids.

What are gonadotrophins?

The pituitary produces two hormones which regulate the gonads, FSH and LH. FSH stimulates the gonads to produce the gametes, ova from the ovary, spermatozoa from the testes. LH is the other gonadotrophin, and it stimulates the gonads to secrete sex hormones, either oestrogen and progesterone from the ovary or testosterone from the testes. In therapeutics LH and FSH can be used to treat some cases of female infertility where ovulation is absent.

Another way of treating infertility due to low gonadotrophin production is to use clomiphene, an estrogen antagonist. It is believed to stimulate FSH and LH release by interfering with the feedback inhibition of estrogen on the pituitary.

What is TSH?

TSH is the trophic hormone from the anterior pituitary which stimulates the thyroid to produce thyroid hormones. Like the gonadotrophins and ACTH, control of TSH is by feedback inhibition by the thyroid hormones thyroxine (T4) and liothyronine (T3). TSH is not used in therapy, as hyperthyroidism is generally due to thyroid failure rather than pituitary failure. TSH assay is important in the diagnosis of neonatal hyperthyroidism which leads to mental retardation or cretinism if undiagnosed. In this condition the failure at thyroid level and hence high TSH levels are present in the blood.

What is GH?

GH is a protein which stimulates growth. Congenital pituitary dwarfism is due to a deficiency of this hormone. Replacement therapy is difficult because GH has not been synthesized and animal GH is not effective in man. The only source of human GH is the human pituitary, and glands are collected at post-mortem in most hospitals and the hormones extracted. GH from hundreds of pituitaries is needed to treat one child with pituitary dwarfism. Oversecretion of GH is usually due to a pituitary tumour. If such a tumour occurs before puberty, giantism is produced and after puberty acromegaly. Pituitary ablation is the treatment of these conditions and not drugs.

What is prolactin?

Prolactin is a hormone whose principal effect is to induce the breast to lactate. Blood levels of prolactin increase 50-fold in pregnancy but the action of prolactin on the breast is blocked by the high circulating levels of oestrogen in the pregnant woman. However, after birth of the child and the placenta, levels of oestrogen fall rapidly and lactation begins. Suppression of lactation can be produced in three ways:

(1) Using no drugs. This leads to breast engorgement and pain but the discomfort is short-lived.

(2) By administering large doses of oestrogen within 24 hours of delivery. This treatment carries a small risk of venous thrombosis.

(3) By use of bromocriptine, a new drug which acts in the pituitary to suppress prolactin secretion. The drug has to be continued for 2 weeks. Bromocriptine is pharmacologically a dopamine agonist.

What about posterior pituitary hormones?

The posterior pituitary is quite different in structure and function from the anterior part of the gland. Two hormones are produced, ADH and oxytocin, both peptides. Oxytocin is important in labour, where it causes contraction of the uterus. Synthetic oxytocin is widely used to initiate and to accelerate labour. It must be given intravenously and the dose has to be carefully regulated. Overdosage of oxytocin leads to rupture of the uterus and stillbirth. In too low a dose no effect is produced. An ingenious device, the Cardiff pump, automatically regulates the rate of oxytocin infusion in labour, basing the dose infused on the intrauterine pressure which is measured via a tube pushed through the cervix and into the uterine cavity.

ADH is a hormone concerned with water balance in the body. It increases reabsorption of water in the renal tubules and hence reduces urine volume. The secretion of ADH is regulated by the osmolarity of the blood; when osmolarity drops ADH secretion is reduced. In the disease diabetes insipidus ADH secretion is defective and patients have a high output of urine. They become dehydrated and thirsty and have to drink large volumes of water. Replacement therapy with ADH is usually effective in this condition and synthetic ADH or an analogue can be given either by nasal spray or by intramuscular depot injection. In one form of the disease, however, the kidney is insensitive to ADH and paradoxically, in this condition, thiazide diuretics are effective at reducing the urine volume.

What about the thyroid gland?

The thyroid produces two hormones which both contain iodine, thyroxine (T4) and liothyronine (T3). These hormones are necessary for growth, for mental development and for metabolic normality. In hypothyroidism the metabolic rate is low and the patient is sluggish and constipated, and the hair and skin show characteristic changes. Hypothyroidism in the developing child leads to mental deficiency or cretinism.

Conversely in hyperthyroidism the patient becomes physically and mentally overactive and has an increased cardiac output.

In hypothyroidism oral synthetic T4 is the effective treatment. It is partially converted in the body to T3 so that the replacement therapy is completely physiological. The maintenance dose in an adult is surprisingly constant in most patients, between 0.1 mg and 0.2 mg/day.

Hyperthyroidism can be treated with a variety of drugs. It is usual to try antithyroid drugs first, and then proceed to surgery or radioiodine treatment if the patient relapses on stopping the antithyroid drugs after 6 months treatment. Antithyroid drugs such as carbimazole and propylthiouracil work by blocking synthesis of T4 and T3 in the thyroid gland.

There is one other hormone produced in the thyroid gland, calcitonin, and this is concerned with the calcium balance. Calcitonin causes the deposition of calcium in bone. It is used in the treatment of Paget's disease.

What hormones does the adrenal gland produce?

The adrenal gland is two glands in one. The adrenal cortex surrounds the adrenal medulla. The cortex is an endocrine gland which produces a number of steroid hormones, while the medulla produces catecholamines under the influence of its sympathetic innervation. The principle medullary hormone is adrenaline.

The steroids produced by the adrenal cortex include aldosterone, hydrocortisone, corticosterone and some small amounts of androgen and oestrogen. In the normal gland the corticosteroids have two types of action: mineralocorticoid and glucocorticoid. The principle mineralocorticoid action, exemplified by aldosterone, is produced through sodium retention by the body; glucocorticoids produce a whole range of metabolic effects. Synthetic adrenal corticosteroids, such as prednisolone or prednisone are used in many diseases. Their principal indications are as replacement therapy for adrenal insufficiency, in immunosuppression and as anti-inflammatory drugs in a variety of conditions. Corticosteroids or steroids, as they are usually called, produce a whole variety of side-effects on long term treatment, and the fate of patients who are condemned to take them for long periods for various diseases is a very sorry one. Corticosteroid side-effects essentially consist of an exaggeration of the metabolic effects of the natural steroids. These include retention of salt, hypertension, osteoporosis, muscle wasting, diabetes, hirsuitism and the characteristic moon face and stretch marks on the skin. Patients on steroids are also more susceptible to infection and the infection may be masked by the anti-inflammatory effect of the drug.

What do the parathyroid glands do?

The parathyroid glands regulate calcium and phosphorus metabolism. The parathyroids produces parathyroid hormone, which increases blood calcium, mobilizing calcium from the bones and increasing renal phosphorous excretion. In hyperparathyroidism there is excess of the hormone and this is treated by surgery. In hypoparathyroidism, parathyroid hormone replacement is not practical and the usual treatment is to use an analogue of vitamin D. The dose must be carefully regulated. Vitamin D works by increasing the absorption of calcium from the alimentary canal.

21

Diabetes mellitus

What is diabetes mellitus?

Diabetes mellitus is a state of chronic high blood glucose level. It is a condition with a high risk of certain complications, including diabetic retinopathy, arterial disease, renal failure, peripheral neuropathies and coma.

What types of diabetes mellitus are there?

There are two clinical types of the condition, best termed insulin dependent and non-insulin dependent diabetes. The first has an onset in youth, while the latter usually occurs in the elderly. In insulin dependent diabetes, otherwise known as juvenile diabetes or type 1 diabetes, the onset is characterized by a fulminant disease with polyuria, polydipsia and intense breakdown of body protein and fat. Non-insulin dependent diabetes, otherwise called maturity onset or senile or type 2 diabetes, usually begins after middle age and is a much less dramatic disease, although the vascular complications can still kill the patient.

What is wrong with the metabolism of diabetic patients?

Diabetics show a defect in blood sugar regulation, which can be characterized by absolute or relative deficiency of the hormone insulin. Insulin is normally produced by the pancreas in response to elevation of blood glucose after a meal. In insulin dependent diabetics there is a near total lack of insulin release after glucose. In non-insulin dependent diabetics there is a relative deficiency, and some of these patients are 'insulin resistant'. This means that although the amount of insulin released is normal, it does not have as much of a hypoglycaemic effect as it should.

What causes diabetes?

Insulin dependent diabetes is most likely caused by a viral infection of the pancreas which only occurs in patients with a genetic susceptibility to the condition. Non-insulin dependent diabetes probably represents an exhaustion of pancreatic insulin production brought about by prolonged over-consumption of carbohydrate.

How is diabetes mellitus treated?

The goal of treatment is to normalize blood glucose as closely as possible. In the short term if blood glucose is controlled then coma from either hyperglycaemia or hypoglycaemia can be avoided. In the long term the more normal the blood glucose, the less progressive are the severe complications of diabetes. Other therapy is directed towards coping with the complications which arise, notably the retinopathy which is the single most common cause of blindness in adults.

How is the blood sugar level controlled?

Blood sugar is controlled with diet, with injections of insulin, and with oral hypoglycaemic drugs.

What is the role of diet in diabetes management?

Diet is still the cornerstone of treatment. Before insulin was introduced in 1921 diet was all the treatment that could be offered to diabetics. Classically, diabetics are given a low carbohydrate diet. There has recently been some dispute about this, and it has been shown that as long as patients take carbohydrate in an unrefined form with a high fibre intake, then they can be allowed more than was previously thought. In this way the patient is not allowed any refined carbohydrate, but is allowed fruit, brown bread, brown rice, brown pasta, etc. The actual amount of carbohydrate in the diet must be kept constant and the patient must take regular meals. If the amount of carbohydrate is not kept constant, then the insulin requirement will vary and blood glucose control will be erratic. In non-insulin dependent patients the same thing applies, with the additional provision that most of these patients are obese and planned gradual weight reduction by diet is part of their treatment. In summary, then, the diet of a diabetic should have no refined carbohydrate, a fixed amount of unrefined carbohydrate, a low fat content and should be kept constant from day to day.

When is insulin used?

Insulin is indispensable in the treatment of type 1 diabetes but is rarely required in type 2 diabetes. Insulin is a peptide hormone which has to be given by injection. There are many different types of insulins of different origin and different duration of action.

How is the insulin dose regulated?

Dietary intake of carbohydrate, insulin dose and the patient's physical activity are all factors in an equation which control blood glucose in the diabetic. When one factor alters then the others have to be changed as well. The medical management is based on establishing a diet which provides enough calories to keep the patient's weight constant, and then the insulin dose is adjusted to maintain blood glucose as near to normal as possible. The trend nowadays is to concentrate on making frequent blood glucose measurements rather than relying on urinary glucose measurement. The problem is that the amount of glucose appearing in the urine varies between patients for any given blood level of glucose, so urine measurements only give an approximate idea of blood glucose values. The actual regime of insulin administration varies widely from centre to centre, but for good blood sugar control in a diabetic insulin must be given twice daily, usually before breakfast and before the main evening meal.

What insulin preparations are available?

The insulins available for treatment are either made from beef or pork pancreas. Beef insulin differs from human insulin in that two amino acids in the molecule are different from that in the human. Pork insulin is more closely similar to human insulin having a difference of only one amino acid. Therefore it is less allergenic, and now highly purified forms of pork insulin are available. They are much more expensive than the traditional insulins but they do have certain advantages. They do not produce fat necrosis at the site of injection, and they provoke the development of fewer antibodies. Hence they can be used for patients who develop insulin resistance and have allergic responses to insulin. Their use is also recommended in pregnant women and in patients with fat necrosis.

Another difference between the insulins is their duration of action. Long duration insulins are used as a single dose of insulin zinc suspension, or biphasic insulin in the morning. This is convenient but probably not ideal. It is more satisfactory to use a mixture of soluble insulin and intermediate insulin twice daily.

How is the dose of insulin measured?

Insulin is standardized biologically, and its strength is quoted in units per ml. Different strengths of insulin exist, either 20, 40 or 80 units/ml, and this is colour coded on the container. Most patients on insulin inject themselves with the drug, using the front of the thigh, the abdomen or the outer side of the arm. Diabetics become proficient at doing this, once they have been instructed in sterile procedures.

What is the treatment of diabetic coma?

There are several types of coma in diabetes, and hyperglycaemic coma in untreated diabetics or patients with infections is the most common. It is essential that the blood glucose level should be measured when a diabetic is found in coma to arrive at the correct diagnosis. The basic treatment of diabetic coma is rehydration with intravenous fluid and treatment with small doses of soluble insulin usually given intravenously for a rapid action.

What types of oral hypoglycaemics are there?

These drugs are of two different sorts, sulphonylureas and biguanides. The sulphonylureas are thought to work by stimulating the pancreas to produce more insulin. Hence they do not work in insulin dependent diabetics who have no insulin reserve in the pancreas. Biguanides act differently. They do not release insulin but they stimulate the uptake of glucose by body tissues. Biguanides can therefore be used in insulin dependent patients.

What sulphonylureas are there?

The most commonly used drugs are chlorpropamide, tolbutamide, glibenclamide and glipizide. Chlorpropamide has a long duration of action and needs to be taken only once a day in a dose of 150/250 mg. Tolbutamide, glibenclamide and glipizide need to be taken three times a day. Complications in their use include hypoglycaemia if the patient misses a meal, rashes and fluid retention.

When are biguanides used?

Biguanides such as metformin and phenformin are now rarely used as they have been shown to precipitate lactic acidosis and hyperosmolar coma, especially in elderly subjects. They are very much drugs of last resort in the treatment of diabetes.

How frequently should diabetics have their eyes checked?

Young diabetics should have their retinas examined by ophthalmoscopy at least once a year. Unfortunately the retinopathy in diabetes can provoke vitreous haemorrhages, so that a patient may pass rapidly from having perfect vision to having a completely blind eye. Therefore the asymptomatic diabetic should have the eyes examined regularly. Appropriate treatment such as laser coagulation of aberrant new vessels is an important part of managing diabetes.

22

Oral contraception

What are the most effective methods of contraception?

The effectiveness of contraceptive methods is expressed as the 'Pearl Index'. This is the number of pregnancies occurring per 100 women-years at risk, one woman-year being 13 menstrual cycles. The Pearl Index for women taking no contraceptive measures is 80, i.e. of 100 women having regular sexual intercourse for one year 80 will become pregnant if no contraception is practised. The Pearl Index for condoms and diaphragms is 10, for intrauterine contraceptive devices 2, and for oral contraceptives 0.7. Thus combined oral contraceptives are the most effective method, and most of the failures using the pill are due to omission of tablets by the users or interactions with other drugs.

What do oral contraceptives consist of?

Oral contraceptives contain two active ingredients, an oestrogen and a progestagen. The absolute amounts and proportion vary from preparation to preparation. Combined oral contraceptives contain both oestrogen and progestagen but progesterone only tablets are also used, the so-called 'mini-pill'.

How are oral contraceptives taken?

Progesterone only preparations are taken continuously, one pill daily. Combined pills are taken in cycles, one tablet being taken each day for 21 days, commencing on the fifth day after the onset of menstruation. At the end of 21 days withdrawal bleeding occurs and the cycle is recommenced.

How do oral contraceptives work?

The combined pill acts by inhibiting ovulation. There is feedback inhibition of the anterior pituitary gonadotrophins, FSH and LH, so that the ovaries are not stimulated to ovulate in women on the pill. With the progesterone only mini-pill, ovulation is not always suppressed and the major effect here is believed to be thickening of the cervical mucous membrane and changes in the uterine endometrium, which becomes unfavourable to implantation of a fertilized ovum. Because of the different mechanism of action the mini-pill is less effective than the combined type.

What complications does the pill produce?

Serious complications are very uncommon. The most important of these is arterial thrombosis presenting as stroke or myocardial infarction. The risk of this is related to the dose of oestrogen and now no pill has a dose of oestrogen greater than the equivalent of 50 μg of ethinylestradiol. Other factors increasing the risk of arterial thrombosis are cigarette smoking, high blood pressure, heart disease and obesity. The incidence of stroke in women on the pill is four times greater than in women not taking the pill. However, the absolute incidence is low, 1 per 5000 women-years, so the risk for each individual woman is very small. However, since some 3.2 million women are taking the pill in the UK today, it can be calculated that 480 women have a stroke every year as a result of taking the pill, resulting in some 100 deaths.

Apart from these serious side-effects of arterial thrombosis, venous thrombosis also occurs, sometimes complicated by pulmonary embolus. This again is rare.

What other unwanted effects are there?

Women on the pill often complain of non-specific side-effects including nausea, weight gain, headache, fatigue and aching veins. These are thought to be oestrogen effects and often wear off within 2 months of starting the pill. Progesterogenic effects include diminished libido, depression, acne and breast tenderness. Two other important side-effects, detection of which requires regular examinations, include hypertension and diabetes. The combined pill is mildly diabetogenic, meaning that it decreases glucose tolerance in women taking it, and may precipitate frank diabetes mellitus in some women who have an inherent tendency to this condition. The mechanism is complex and not clearly worked out. Women who develop high blood pressure on the pill are believed to do so because the pill stimulates the production of renin substrate in the liver. This is a protein acted upon in the blood by renin, an enzyme produced by the kidney. The result of this action is angiotensin II, a circulating substance which raises the blood pressure.

Are there any women for whom the pill is not suitable?

Yes, women with high blood pressure and previous history of stroke or pulmonary embolus should not be given the pill. Likewise, women with liver disease or sickle cell anaemia, a condition more common in the negroid and Mediterranean population, have a high risk of complications on the pill and should not be given this treatment.

What drugs can interact with oral contraceptives?

Oral contraceptives are metabolized in the liver. In women who are treated with drugs which speed up hepatic metabolism, so-called 'enzyme inducers' contraceptive efficacy from the pill can be lost. Such drugs include barbiturates and certain antibiotics. An indication of this effect is the onset of breakthrough bleeding in mid-cycle, which indicates that the dosage of the pill has fallen too low.

How is the choice of oral contraceptive made?

Oral contraceptives differ in only two ways, the dose of oestrogen and the dose of progestagen. The greater the oestrogen content, then the more effective the contraceptive effect, but the greater the risk of diabetes and thrombosis. Patients complaining of nausea and breast symptoms can sometimes have relief of these symptoms by moving to a lower dose oestrogen pill. However, the room for manoeuvre with oestrogen dosage is rather small now that the highest dose of oestrogen is 50 μg for ethinylestradiol. There are in fact only pills containing 50 and 30 μg of ethinylestradiol on the market, and of course the mini-pill which contains no oestrogen at all. Progesterone content of combined pills varies more widely from the equivalent of 1 mg of norethisterone up to 4 mg. As progesterone content is increased depression, weight gain and fatigue are increasingly complained of.

What about the progesterone only mini-pill?

The mini-pill only containing progesterone is a less effective oral contraceptive than the combined pill, but is still more effective than an intrauterine contraceptive device. It is principally used by women to whom it is thought unwise to give any dose of oestrogen namely those who have some history of cardiovascular trouble. It is also suitable for women who are older and who have a lower fertility. The problem with the mini-pill is that it is taken continuously and in some women the cycle length or frequency of menstruation may be short.

What is a triphasic pill?

Triphasic pills are a recent innovation in which the doses of progestagen and oestrogen are varied at different phases of the menstrual cycle so as to mimic normal hormone patterns more closely. The progestagen dose increases through the month, 50 μg for the first 6 days, 75 μg for the next 5 days and 125 μg for the last 10 days. The oestrogen dose is 30 μg daily except during the middle 5 days when it is 40 μg. The theoretical advantage of such a complex dosing scheme over a fixed-dose combination is that the total dose of progestagen can be lower without loss of efficacy. In practice triphasic pills may be a good choice for those women at particular risk from cardiovascular side-effects, such as older women and smokers.

23

Drugs and pregnancy

What drugs are used in pregnancy?

The average pregnant woman takes more than four different drugs during the course of her pregnancy. About half of these are taken during the first 3 months, when there is a risk of teratogenesis.

What is teratogenesis?

Teratogenesis is the production of a congenital abnormality by some external agency such as a drug, radiation or viral infection.

How common is teratogenesis?

About 2% of all babies born in the UK have a congenital malformation, although many of these are of a minor nature. The cause of most of these congenital malformations is not known. Certain infections have been identified as teratogenic. The best known of these is german measles which can cause multiple congenital lesions if the mother contracts it in early pregnancy. About 10% of all congenital abnormalities have been ascribed to the teratogenic effects of drugs taken in the critical period early in pregnancy when embryogenesis and organogenesis is taking place. This corresponds to the period up to 8 weeks after conception. However this figure of 10% is a rough estimate and all that is really known about the role of drugs in teratogenesis is the following:

(1) Many drugs and chemicals cause congenital abnormalities if given to animals at a critical stage of pregnancy.

(2) Some drugs have been proved to cause congenital abnormalities in human babies. This list is short.

(3) Many drugs are taken in early pregnancy, so that there is at least a possibility of them being able to induce a congenital abnormality.

What drugs are teratogenic in man?

Realization that drugs could be teratogenic in human pregnancy is relatively recent. It dates from the thalidomide disaster in the early 1960s. Prior to that time the fetus was thought to be insulated from drug effects by its separate circulation and the placenta. Thalidomide is certainly highly teratogenic, a single dose of this sleeping tablet being sufficient to cause abnormality if taken at the critical stage in the pregnancy. No other drug of similar potency has been identified and it is believed that thalidomide is a unique case. However, some drugs are thought to be minor teratogens as follows:

(1) Cytotoxic drugs of all sorts. It is obvious that a drug which attacks dividing cells will be particularly toxic to the embryo, and it is known from occasions when cytotoxic drugs have been taken by women who are trying to procure an abortion that these substances can cause congenital abnormalities. In the normal course of events it would be extremely rare for a woman to be taking these drugs during pregnancy, although they are occasionally used as part of immunosuppressive regimes in women with transplants who have become pregnant. Azathioprine has been taken in pregnancy on several occasions in this circumstance, and surprisingly has produced no congenital abnormalities.

(2) Anticonvulsant drugs. The incidence of congenital abnormalities in women with epilepsy who have taken anticonvulsants is slightly higher than in the general population, and several anticonvulsants are teratogenic in animals.

(3) Tetracycline. If tetracycline is taken at any stage of the pregnancy it can cause staining of the teeth and bones in the child so exposed. This is obviously not a disastrous malformation, but tetracycline should be avoided in pregnant women and children.

(4) Sex hormones. These should be avoided in pregnancy as they can interfere with sexual differentiation, and one hormone stilboestrol, an oestrogen, has been shown to produce cancer in the children of women treated with it during pregnancy.

(5) Vitamin D in high doses. This vitamin has been associated with congenital heart abnormalities in the babies of women who have taken it in high doses during pregnancy.

How are drugs determined to be teratogenic in man?

Since the thalidomide disaster, all drugs have been tested for teratogenic effects on at least two different species of animals. Unfortunately every species has a different sensitivity to teratogenic drugs, and it is known that some drugs which are teratogenic in animals are harmless in man. An example of this would be aspirin and caffeine which are teratogenic in some rodents but not in man. Conversely, thalidomide, the most potent teratogen in man, is not teratogenic in many animal species and even in primates larger doses have to be given than in man to produce the effect. Therefore, animal tests are only a rough guide to fetal and embryonic toxicity, and they do not actually predict what will happen in human pregnancy.

For these reasons new drugs are not given to pregnant women, at least in early pregnancy, unless it is absolutely essential. However, it is inevitable, that over the years pregnant women will receive a drug either in error or because the use is essential, or because women become pregnant who are already taking the drug, or the drug is given to women who do not know they are pregnant when they receive it. The case records of all these exposures add to our knowledge on the safety or danger of the drug in pregnancy. Obviously this is not a very satisfactory system but unless the biochemical mechanisms underlying teratogenesis are worked out, then the situation is not likely to change.

How does teratogenicity come about?

Teratogenesis is an example of selective toxicity of the sort already discussed in the chapters on chemotherapy. The drug is toxic to one individual, the embryo or fetus, and not to the host mother. Why this selectivity occurs is not well worked out. One explanation is to relate it to the increased rate of cell division in the conceptus, which become susceptible to the toxic effects of drugs acting at cell division. Hence the sensitivity to cytotoxics. Another explanation is that the embryo has a different circulatory system to the mother, and clears drugs less rapidly than the maternal circulation. This could lead to accumulation of the drug and a relatively high dose in the fetus. Another factor is the different capacity of fetal tissue to metabolize the drug. There is often a different pattern of metabolites produced in the fetus compared with the mother. In this way reactive toxic metabolites, such as epoxides, can be formed in the fetus and be less rapidly broken down than they are in the adult. Such reactive intermediates can bind to nuclear proteins and cause mutations. Lastly, the fetus may be particularly susceptible to the effect of sex hormones since these normally control differentiation of sexual organs within the fetus. The presence of exogenous sex steroids is likely to upset normal sexual development.

What can be done about drug teratogenicity?

It is easy to say that the problem of drug teratogenicity can be dealt with by the complete avoidance of drug exposure in pregnant women, at least during the first 3 months. However, there are problems to enforcing this. Women may not realize they are pregnant until after the critical phase has passed. Some women certainly require long term medical treatment, which it would be hazardous to stop. Intercurrent illness may require drug treatment during the pregnancy. Finally, there are specific conditions which occur during the course of pregnancy which require treatment, such as hypertension and intrauterine growth retardation of the fetus. Here increasingly drug treatment will be used. The problem of potential teratogenicity is a difficult one but it should be kept in proportion; the vast majority of drugs to which the woman is exposed are not likely to harm the pregnancy.

What about the use of drugs in labour?

Two main types of drugs are used in labour, oxytocics and analgesics. Labour can be induced with an intravenous infusion of oxytocin or with the use of prostaglandins. Prostaglandin E_2 is the most commonly used. This is a naturally occurring substance which is believed to be involved in the initiation of normal labour. It can be used intravenously but causes less diarrhoea and vomiting if it is instilled directly on to the cervix as a pessary or a paste. Acceleration of a poorly progressive labour is best carried out with an oxytocin infusion, but the dose of this infusion has to be carefully regulated to avoid uterine hypertonus.

Analgesia in labour is a specialized subject. The trend nowadays is towards more use of epidural analgesia. In this technique a local anaesthetic is infused via a catheter placed in the epidural space of the lower back, allowing selective anaesthesia of the sensory innervation of the cervix and vagina. It is even possible to use this technique for caesarean section, so that the mother is conscious during the operation. More conventional analgesia in labour includes intravenous and intramuscular opiates and inhalational drugs such as nitrous oxide, oxygen and Trilene mixtures. A particular hazard of general anaesthetics in labour is the inhalation of vomit which can be fatal. The hazards of analgesia in labour include depression of the fetus, so that it is in poor condition to breathe and suckle after birth.

Why are drugs taken in early pregnancy?

About half the exposures to drugs in early pregnancy are a result of 'over-the-counter' purchases, such drugs as analgesics, antacids, aspirins and cold cures forming the bulk of the exposures. The use of cold cures is probably the most worrying. Most of these remedies contain, as their active ingredient, a sympathomimetic amine having a pharmacology similar to ephedrine, which acts to relieve nasal congestion by constricting the blood vessels in the nose. Unfortunately, some surveys have shown that such amines are teratogenic in man, causing limb deformation and they should not be used by women who are or who might be pregnant.

What about prescribed drugs?

The most commonly used drugs in pregnancy are antibiotics for incidental infections and maintenance therapy for medical conditions such as hypertension or epilepsy. In all these cases the possible risk of teratogenesis must be weighed against clinical benefit. With the exception of tetracycline and trimethoprim most antibiotics are thought to be quite safe for pregnant women to take. Almost all pregnant women are given iron tablets in pregnancy, often in combination with folic acid. There is no evidence that such treatment is harmful to the fetus and the incidence of anaemia in pregnancy is thereby reduced.

What about drugs for morning sickness?

Antihistamines, vitamins and phenothiazine drugs are all effective treatments for the nausea many women experience in early pregnancy. There is no evidence to suggest that such drugs are teratogenic but morning sickness is usually a trivial condition which passes as the pregnancy progresses and no drug treatment is necessary. Many women prefer to put up with morning sickness rather than take any drug which might be deleterious to the baby.

What about drugs after the delivery?

Analgesia is often required for perineal pain especially if an episiotomy has been done. Drugs which influence breast feeding are often given. Lactation can be suppressed with bromocriptine, a dopamine agonist which is discussed in Chapter 20 on endocrinology.

SECTION 6

THE KIDNEY AND THE GUT

24

Diuretics and the kidney

What are diuretics?

Diuresis means the production of urine. Hence, diuretics are substances whose administration increases urine production. However, this strict definition certainly includes water so a more practical definition of a diuretic is a drug which increases the renal excretion of salt and water.

When are diuretics used?

Diuretics are used in the treatment of hypertension as previously discussed, and in the treatment of salt and water retention. Salt and water retention often manifests as oedema, which occurs in three situations: cardiac failure, hepatic failure and the nephrotic syndrome. In heart failure, oedema occurs because of poor perfusion of the kidney, and because of back pressure of blood in the capillaries leading exudation of fluid. In liver disease albumin synthesis is decreased and hence the osmotic pressure of blood falls, allowing transudation of fluid into the tissues. The nephrotic syndrome is a kidney disease where large amounts of protein are lost in the urine. This reduces blood albumin, again leading to oedema.

What diuretics are there?

There are three main groups of diuretics: the thiazides, the loop diuretics and the potassium sparing diuretics. Other, now obsolete, drugs with diuretic action include the mercurial diuretics and the osmotic diuretics.

How do diuretics work?

The daily urinary output in a normal adult is between 1–2 litres. This represents about 1% of the fluid which the kidney skims off the blood in the kidney glomeruli and passes down the renal tubules. Most of the filtrate is reabsorbed. Diuretic drugs interfere with this reabsorption in the renal tubules (Figure 12) and allow more salt and water to be excreted. Diuretic drugs do not actively cause water and salt to be excreted. They merely interfere with the normal conservation process in the kidney and allow more salt and water to be lost.

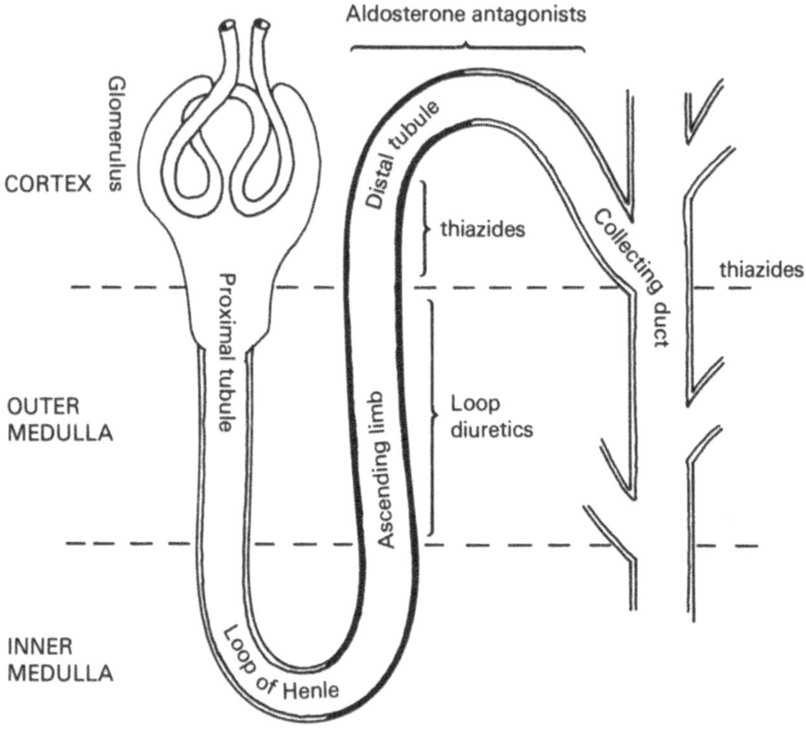

Figure 12 Anatomy of a renal tubule showing where some types of diuretic drugs act

What are the thiazide diuretics?

Thiazides are the standard oral diuretics first introduced into practice in 1958. There are many of them, chlorothiazide, bendrofluazide, cyclopenthiazide, etc. and they have very similar actions and side-effects. These drugs interfere with sodium reabsorption from a distal part of the renal tubule. As a result of their action the urine contains more salt and more potassium.

When are thiazides used?

They are used in hypertension and as a first-line treatment of cardiac failure, cirrhosis of the liver and nephrotic syndrome. In severe oedema and intractable heart failure the thiazides are replaced by the more potent loop diuretics.

What are the loop diuretics?

Loop diuretics are drugs which act to prevent sodium absorption at more sites in the tubules than the thiazide diuretics. They are active both in the proximal and in the distal tubules and also in the loop of Henle (which is that part of the nephron which dips into the medulla of the kidney and where most concentration of the urine occurs). As a result of these multiple sites of action, the loop diuretics are more powerful than the thiazides and produce more salt and water loss. The most commonly used drug is frusemide, but ethacrynic acid and bumetanide have similar actions. These drugs are no more useful than thiazides in hypertension but are reserved for intractable oedema. In addition loop diuretics are useful in the acute treatment of left ventricular failure where fluid is being spilled from the blood into the lungs. Here the drug is given intravenously and is rapidly effective.

What are the side-effects of thiazides and loop diuretics?

All these diuretics cause potassium depletion and are often given together with potassium supplements or with drugs which selectively conserve potassium. Whether potassium depletion is important or not is disputed but it certainly matters in patients who are taking digitalis. Other complications of diuretic therapy include the precipitation of diabetes mellitus and gout. The diuretics compete with uric acid for excretion by the renal tubules and this is how they cause gout. Over-usage of powerful diuretics can sometimes cause dehydration and salt depletion.

What are the potassium sparing diuretics?

These drugs are often used in combination with thiazides to prevent potassium loss. They are of two sorts. Amiloride and triamterene are similar drugs which cause potassium retention by the distal tubule, together with an increased excretion of uric acid. They are thus useful drugs to be used in combination with thiazides, and combinations of tablets are widely used in the treatment of hypertension.

Spironolactone is a drug with a different action. It competitively antagonizes the effect of aldosterone on the renal tubules. Aldosterone is the adrenal corticosterone hormone which causes sodium retention and potassium loss by the kidney. Secretion of this hormone is found to be increased in cirrhosis of the liver and in cardiac failure, exacerbating the tendency to salt and water retention. In these patients spironolactone is an effective drug causing salt and water loss and retention of potassium. In renal failure there is a failure of potassium excretion and potassium sparing diuretics are hazardous in such patients.

25

Drugs and the digestive system

What drugs are available for gastrointestinal problems?

Drugs for gastrointestinal problems are among the most commonly prescribed medicines. Gut motility can be controlled by drugs leading to effective therapy for diarrhoea or constipation. Drugs acting on the vomiting centre of the brain can induce or relieve nausea and vomiting. Acid secretion by the stomach is another important target of drug action. The acid can be neutralized with alkalis, and very recently drugs have been introduced which can selectively reduce acid secretion by the stomach providing an effective treatment against peptic ulcer.

What is dyspepsia and how is it treated?

Dyspepsia or indigestion means different things to different patients. It can be loosely defined as abdominal pain or discomfort related to meals. For many dyspepsia is merely the occasional sequel of overindulgence and responds to a proprietary antacid tablet. In patients with occasional dyspepsia if the stomach is examined by gastroscope during an attack, the most common finding is reddening of the stomach antrum and oesophagus. Persistent habitual dyspepsia requires investigation, and the commonest causes of this syndrome are gastro-oesophagal reflux due to hiatus hernia, duodenal or gastric ulcer or gallstones. Each of these has a distinctive symptom complex.

What causes duodenal ulcers?

Duodenal ulcers are common. About 5% of men have one at some time in their lives. They usually affect young individuals living a stressed and hurried existence. Smoking cigarettes is a contributory cause. Duodenal ulcers only occur in the presence of an acid secreting mucosa, and patients with established duodenal ulcers have been shown to have a greater acid production than normal.

How is a duodenal ulcer treated?

The treatment has changed in recent years with the introduction of cimetidine, the first of a new class of drugs which directly inhibit the secretion of acid by the stomach. Prior to this discovery the only therapies proven to be effective in healing ulcers were bed rest, stopping smoking and treatment with carbonoxolone, a drug derived from liquorice. However, none of these treatments was very effective and the relapse rate was high. Many duodenal ulcer patients eventually came to surgery, undergoing operations designed to cut the capacity of the stomach to secrete acid. It must be noted, however, that the natural history of duodenal ulcer is a relapsing one with periods of exacerbation and healing. Apart from the treatments designed to heal the ulcer, a number of measures are known to give relief from the symptoms, particularly the use of antacids and frequent small meals. Both antacids and food neutralize gastric acid.

How does cimetidine work?

It has been known for a very long time that patients with duodenal ulcers have an excessive secretion of gastric acid. Ingestion of food is the physiological stimulus which provokes the release of acid from the stomach. The hormone gastrin is produced by the mucosa of the stomach and duodenum, and acts on the stomach to provoke the release of gastric acid. Intermediate in the action of gastrin is the release of the hormone histamine in the stomach. Histamine has many different actions in the body, including vasodilatation, increased permeability of blood vessels and stimulation of gastric acid secretion. All the actions of histamine, apart from gastric secretion, can be blocked by antihistamines, drugs which have been available for many years and are used in the treatment of allergy and hay fever where histamine plays a part. It is only recently that drugs have been developed which antagonize the gastric effect of histamine. This dual action of histamine has been explained on the basis of histamine activating different sorts of receptors in different tissues, so-called H_1-receptors in the blood vessels and skin which are blocked by antihistamine drugs, and H_2-receptors in the stomach.

Cimetidine, the first H_2-receptor blocker, has been shown to inhibit gastric acid secretion in response to most stimuli. As might be expected, this drug is very effective at healing duodenal ulcers. Cimetidine is used in the dose 200 mg three times a day with meals, and 400 mg at night. Using this regime about 60% of duodenal ulcers heal within 6 weeks. Symptomatic relief occurs almost immediately the treatment is begun, because it is the acid which causes the ulcer pain. Unfortunately some patients relapse if the cimetidine treatment is stopped because, of course, the factors which provoke the ulcer in the first place may still be operating. Surgery still has a place in the treatment of a duodenal ulcer which is intractable or recurrent. It is still important that the patient should stop smoking. Side-effects of cimetidine are infrequent, but they include diarrhoea, skin rashes and confusion, especially in elderly patients.

What about gastric ulcers?

Gastric ulcers arise in a different way from duodenal ulcers. They occur more commonly in the elderly and badly fed individuals, and tend to run a more chronic course. However, like duodenal ulcers, pain from the ulcer occurs because of acid secretion, and cimetidine treatment, which abolishes the secretion of acid, is effective in treating gastric ulcers.

How is gastric reflux treated?

Oesophagitis due to gastric reflux usually occurs in middle aged individuals who are overweight. The management includes weight loss and raising the head of the bed to avoid acid running into the oesophagus at night. Antacids which neutralize gastric acid relieve the pain or heart burn of gastric reflux.

How do antacids work?

Antacids are simply chemical substances which neutralize the hydrochloric acid secreted in the stomach. They are amongst the most widely used medicines, and there are many different preparations available. Any antacid will relieve ulcer pain or dyspepsia if given frequently and in large quantities. The problem is that some antacids are absorbed from the gut and can cause alkalosis. Other antacids are not absorbed but cause constipation. Still others cause diarrhoea in some patients. What is probably most important about an antacid is to select one that the patient finds acceptable and pleasant to take.

The usual ingredients of antacid mixtures include sodium bicarbonate, which can rapidly neutralize gastric acid but releases carbon dioxide causing belching. If it is absorbed in large quantities it can cause alkalosis. Magnesium oxide and carbonate are salts which are not absorbed from the gut and do not provoke alkalosis. However, by remaining in the gut they form a saline purge leading to looseness of the bowels. Calcium carbonate, on the other hand, leads to constipation. Therefore, blending these various salts is worthwhile, and mixtures of magnesium and calcium carbonate can be effective antacids without upsetting bowel function. Other popular antacid salts are magnesium trisilicate which may also provoke some diarrhoea, and aluminium hydroxide, another salt with a good antacid action but with an astringent action which can provoke constipation. Proprietary antacids usually contain a mixture of all these substances with some flavouring. In general, antacids are effective at relieving dyspepsia though the action is not very long lasting.

What other drugs are used for the treatment of gastric and duodenal ulcer?

Drugs which block the vagus nerve also interfere with gastric secretion though they are much less effective than H_2 blockers (p. 140). Atropine-like drugs, such as poldine, have been used for this action for many years, but have now been superseded by the H_2 blockers. Their side-effects include dry mouth and interference with ocular accommodation.

What drugs can cause gastric bleeding?

A variety of drugs can provoke gastric bleeding. Corticosteroids can induce gastric and duodenal ulceration or reactivate a healed ulcer. Since some anticoagulants can provoke gastric or gastrointestinal bleeding, the presence of an active or recently healed duodenal ulcer is certainly a contraindication of these drugs. However, the most common groups of drugs provoking gastric bleeding are the non-steroidal anti-inflammatory drugs (NSAID) used as mild analgesics, and anti-inflammatories, of which aspirin is the most common. Most patients on chronic aspirin therapy suffer from very mild gastric bleeding which is of little consequence. However, ingestion of aspirin can occasionally provoke a brisk bleed, and if such patients are investigated soon after the event, multiple erosions may be seen in the stomach.

What treatment is there for gallstones?

Until recently the only treatment for gall stones was surgical removal of the gall bladder. However, the pathology of gall stone formation has become recently clearer. Most gall stones consist of cholesterol, and it has been shown that patients forming these stones do so because their bile is deficient in bile salts. Oral administration of the synthetic bile salt chenodeoxycholic acid can cause dissolution of these cholesterol gall-stones if the salt is taken for a period of months. The treatment must be prolonged and its place in the management of gall stones has yet to be assessed. Unfortunately once the treatment is discontinued the patient's bile reverts to its cholesterol saturated state.

What drugs can be used as anti-nauseants?

Vomiting is a complex act initiated and controlled not by the stomach but by a vomiting centre in the hind brain. Vomiting can be induced by drugs such as apomorphine, which stimulate the vomiting centre. Conversely, nausea and vomiting can be antagonized by drugs which have a depressing effect on the vomiting centre. There are a number of these drugs which can be divided into three types: antihistamines, phenothiazines and metoclopramide. Most antihistamines have an antiemetic action. Cyclizine is an antihistamine which is an effective antinauseant when given orally or intramuscularly. It is particularly effective at antagonizing the nausea and vomiting produced by opiate drugs, and is often given with these to prevent post-operative vomiting. Among the phenothiazines, chlorpromazine or perphenazine are powerful antiemetics, and they can also be given orally or by injection. Finally, metoclopramide is an anti-emetic which probably also has a peripheral action causing a more rapid emptying of the stomach into the duodenum. The dose of metoclopramide is 10 mg three times a day; it is also used in the treatment of dyspepsia because of its peripheral action.

What about nausea in pregnancy?

Nausea is characteristic of early pregnancy and must be regarded as a normal event. The cause is not known. Occasionally the nausea and vomiting progresses to such a point that the patient becomes ill and begins to lose weight. This condition is known as hyperemesis gravidarum and necessitates admission to hospital and intravenous feeding. However, in most cases morning sickness is mild and can be partially alleviated by giving the patient something to eat and drink before she gets out of bed in the morning. Antihistamines are effective at preventing morning sickness and there is no good evidence that they can harm the developing embryo and fetus. Nevertheless, the doubt hangs over any drug used in early pregnancy. Most women will be prepared to put up with mild symptoms of nausea in early pregnancy to avoid the slightest chance of any teratogenic effect.

What causes constipation?

Constipation is a disturbance of colonic function. The usual cause is dietary. The modern Western diet contains a high proportion of refined foods with little bulk or cellulose. Because of this little residual material enters the colon and as the colon absorbs water from the bowel contents, the stool becomes hard and small. As a result, the small stool does not distend the rectum and the characteristic sensation of a full rectum is not felt. In the past, this sequence of events was not really appreciated and the usual response to complaints of constipation was to recommend the use of purgatives rather than alteration of the diet. It is now felt that purgatives should be seen as drugs only for occasional use, e.g. in preparation of the bowel for surgery or barium examination.

What types of purgative are there?

Purgatives can be classified into three types: irritant purges, bulk purgatives and emollient purgatives. Irritants increase bowel peristalsis, allowing less water to be absorbed. Bulk purgatives consist of unabsorbable material which swells the intestinal contents; cellulose or agar agar is often used. Emollient purgatives consist of mineral oils, which are also not absorbed, and alter the consistency of the gut contents.

SECTION 7
THE BLOOD

26

Drugs and anaemia

What drugs are used in the treatment of anaemia?

There are many different causes of anaemia and a precise diagnosis should be made before treatment is started. However, most anaemias are due to a deficiency of dietary factors used in the synthesis of red cells. These deficiencies can be remedied by treatment with haematinics, which are drugs that stimulate blood production. The most important of these haematinics is iron.

How does iron deficiency anaemia occur?

Patients can become iron deficient either because of loss of blood or because their diet is deficient in iron. Patients presenting with anaemia shown to be due to iron deficiency must be investigated to exclude blood loss, particularly occult blood loss from the gut. Gastrointestinal tumours, ulcers or simple haemorrhoids are common causes.

The daily requirement of iron in normal adults is around 1 mg/day for men, 1.5 mg for premenopausal women and 3.5 mg for pregnant women. A normal diet contains around 10 mg of iron per day, but the absorption of iron from the gut is selective and only 10% is normally absorbed. However, if iron deficiency occurs, then up to 30% of the dietary iron can be absorbed as a result of the body's adaptation. Where the diet consists mainly of cereals iron is less easily absorbed from the gut.

It can be seen from this account that balance between the iron in the diet and what is required by the body is rather critical. It is quite possible for people to become iron deficient even on what appears to be a reasonable diet. This is particularly true of premenopausal women because of their increased iron losses. Therefore, iron deficiency is relatively common. Surveys in this country have shown that evidence of iron deficiency can be found in about one-fifth of all women before the menopause.

What sort of problems does iron deficiency cause?

The blood picture in iron deficiency anaemia is hypochromic, that is the red cells contain less haemoglobin than usual. Other clinical features include cracking at the corners of the mouth, a smooth tongue and difficulty with swallowing. In severe anaemia there can be breathlessness on exertion.

How is iron deficiency treated?

In most cases an iron deficiency can be treated with oral iron. Occasionally in patients who do not respond, iron can be given intramuscularly or even intravenously. There is a definite hazard to giving iron in this way including anaphylactic reactions, so that the oral route is much preferred.

Iron is given orally in the form of a ferrous salt in a dose of between 100 and 200 mg a day. This allows the absorption, in somebody who is iron deficient, of around 30 mg/day. Various salts are available and there are many different preparations of iron. The three main ones are tablets of ferrous sulphate, ferrous gluconate, and ferrous fumarate All of these iron preparations have some undesirable side-effects in up to a fifth of all people treated. Constipation and diarrhoea are the commonest side-effects. Oral iron therapy makes the stool a black colour and this sometimes alarms patients. Another very important consideration with iron tablets is that they are poisonous when taken in overdosage. An all too frequent tragedy is that the young children of women being treated with iron tablets mistake them for sweets as many of the proprietary capsules are highly coloured. Iron poisoning in children is an emergency which must be treated in hospital with the administration of desferrioxamine, a drug which binds iron. Without specialist treatment children who take an overdose of iron tablets can die of cardiovascular collapse and anuria.

What other haematinics are there?

Two other important dietary haematinics are folic acid and vitamin B_{12}. Folic acid is a vitamin widely available in the diet particularly in fresh foods. It is necessary for the proper maturation of red cells, and if there is dietary deficiency of this substance the blood shows the changes of macrocytosis, deformed large red cells with anaemia. Folic acid deficiency occurs either because of dietary deficiency or because of malabsorption or occasionally during pregnancy. The diagnosis can be proved biochemically and folic acid can be given either orally or intramuscularly.

What about vitamin B_{12}?

Deficiency of vitamin B_{12} leads to pernicious anaemia. This is not due to dietary deficiency of vitamin B_{12} but to a failure of absorption of the vitamin from the small intestine. The vitamin is not absorbed because of a deficiency of intrinsic factor in the stomach. Pernicious anaemia apparently results from atrophy of the stomach and is probably an autoimmune disease. Treatment of the anaemia is by parenteral administration of the vitamin, injections being given at least monthly.

27

Anticoagulation

What are anticoagulants?

Anticoagulants are drugs which interfere with the blood clotting mechanism. The normal clotting of blood is a complex sequential process, one plasma protein being activated to cleave another and so on in a cascade until the final protein, fibrinogen, is split to yield fibrin. Fibrin is the protein which meshes the blood cells into a blood clot. Thrombosis occurring inside a blood vessel is a somewhat different process, primarily involving blood platelets aggregating together to form a solid jelly-like clump. This subsequently induces blood to clot around it.

What anticoagulants are there?

There are two types of anticoagulant, oral anticoagulants and heparin, and they act in completely different ways.

How do oral anticoagulants work?

The synthesis of certain proteins involved in clotting is dependent upon the availability of vitamin K in the liver where the proteins are made. The oral anticoagulants are competitive antagonists of vitamin K and slow down the production of these proteins. The result is that the blood plasma contains less of these clotting factors, the blood clots more slowly and the bleeding time is prolonged. The dose of oral anticoagulants is crucial; if too much drug is taken spontaneous haemorrhage will occur. Oral anticoagulant drugs are also used as rat poisons.

What is heparin?

Heparin is a natural substance which occurs in the lung and liver. The drug is extracted from beef lung. Its action is to interfere with the conversion of fibrinogen to fibrin and heparin can completely prevent the clotting of blood. It is used to keep blood specimens liquid. In therapy heparin has to be given by intravenous injection as it is not absorbed by mouth. The action of heparin is immediate and wears off rapidly so it has to be given by continuous infusion or at least by 6 hourly injection. Heparin can be given subcutaneously but it causes bruising.

When are anticoagulants used?

Anticoagulants are used to treat thrombosis. Unfortunately they are rather unsuccessful in the treatment of arterial thrombosis which is the underlying problem in coronary thrombosis, thrombotic stroke and peripheral gangrene. Their relative inefficacy in arterial thrombosis is probably because thrombosis is mainly a platelet-mediated event rather than true blood clotting. However, anticoagulants are effective in treating and preventing venous thrombosis, which can lead to pulmonary embolus. Heparin is a very useful drug in extracorporeal circulations which are used increasingly frequently in modern medicine. Such procedures as renal dialysis, heart lung bypass or artificial liver perfusions could not be carried out if heparin were not added to the blood in order to prevent clotting in the machines.

How are oral anticoagulants used?

Warfarin or phenindione is the drug usually chosen. Phenindione has a shorter halflife of 5 hours whereas warfarin is longer acting with a halflife of 44 hours. Therefore, warfarin is given once a day and phenindione 3 times a day. These drugs do not anticoagulate directly, and their effect only comes on once the effect of decreased synthesis of clotting factors has taken effect; hence anticoagulation is not produced until 24 hours after dosing. The dose of each drug must be adjusted according to the prothrombin time, which is a test giving an indication of by how much clotting factors in blood have been reduced. Initially, the prothrombin time must be measured frequently until a stable anti-coagulant dose is obtained. Thereafter, blood tests in patients on a stable dose can be repeated at monthly intervals.

What are the adverse effects of oral anticoagulants?

All anticoagulants are hazardous, and do have a high incidence of adverse effects, the most important being bleeding and bruising. If bleeding is severe, then the effect of the drugs can be completely reversed by giving vitamin K. Allergic side-effects are also seen, fewer with warfarin than with phenindione.

What precautions are necessary for a patient on oral anticoagulants?

Patients should be warned to report all incidents of bleeding, to avoid injury and violent exercise and not to undergo dental extractions, except in hospital. They should not take any other drugs while on anti-coagulants, except those which have been prescribed by the doctor controlling the anticoagulation. Many other drugs interact with the oral anticoagulants, either potentiating or diminishing their effect and this can have serious consequences.

How do drug interactions with the anticoagulants occur?

There are many interactions but three, in particular, are important. If a patient on anticoagulants takes antibiotics then the supply of vitamin K synthesized in the gut by bacteria may fall, and the anticoagulant can have an exaggerated effect leading to bleeding. Secondly, drugs such as phenylbutazone can provoke bleeding because they displace the drug from binding to plasma protein and temporarily increase its circulating free concentration. Finally, inducing agents such as barbiturate sleeping tablets can enhance warfarin metabolism, and if they are stopped suddenly then the rebound decrease in warfarin metabolism can lead to increased drug effects and more bleeding.

Are there any patients who should not be given anticoagulants?

There are several conditions where there is a tendency to bleeding. Patients with high blood pressure may develop a cerebral haemorrhage, patients who have had surgery may bleed from the wound, and patients with duodenal and gastric ulcers are at risk of haemorrhage. Anti-coagulants should not be given to such patients.

What about antiplatelet agents?

There has been a lot of research recently on the way in which platelets aggregate together to form a thrombus. It is now known that one of the most active antiplatelet drugs is aspirin, which prevents the formation inside the platelet of a prostaglandin, thromboxane, which is necessary for the platelets to aggregate. Other drugs with a more specific effect on the thromboxane system are being developed, and there is some hope that antiplatelet drugs can be developed which are effective in prevent-ing the important conditions of coronary thrombosis and cerebral thrombosis. Furthermore, there is some evidence that arterial disease occurs secondarily to disorders of platelets which stick on to blood vessel walls and induce atheroma. Since just under half of all deaths in the UK are a direct consequence of arterial disease or arterial throm-bosis, these are important matters on which there has been relatively little progress in the past. Of particular interest is the pharmacology of a new recently discovered prostaglandin, called prostacyclin. This substance is synthesized by blood vessel walls, and apparently normally inhibits platelets from sticking to the normal blood vessel walls. If the prostacyclin synthetase system is deranged, as is believed to happen in atheroma, then intramural thrombosis can occur. Drugs which mimic prostacyclin activity are a possible approach to this problem, but are as yet in the experimental stage.

SECTION 8

TOPICAL THERAPY

28

Drugs and the skin

What is topical therapy?

Many different drugs can be applied directly to the skin in the form of ointments, creams or sprays. When drugs are applied locally, as in treating skin diseases, this is called *topical therapy*. However, drugs are often absorbed when rubbed onto the skin and can then have a systemic effect. Such generalized effects are usually an unwanted nuisance, an example being the suppression of adrenal function when steroid creams are used. Occasionally, however, skin application of a drug is used to provide a rapid and sustained effect. For example, glyceryl trinitrate ointment can relieve angina when rubbed onto the chest. 'Strap-on drugs' have been developed where the drug diffuses out of the plaster and into the skin, to provide a more sustained effect than when a single tablet is swallowed. Such new approaches may be useful, but will probably be limited by the development of local allergy to the drug.

How are drugs applied to the skin?

Drugs for topical uses are mixed with semi-liquid pastes to make them easy to apply. *Ointments* are greasy and are not miscible with water. *Creams* are emulsions formed from water and oil and are more easily washed off. *Pastes* are the thickest form of applications, and are useful for fixing drugs to small discrete areas. *Lotions* are dispersions of drugs in water which dry after application leaving a powder on the skin.

How are some of the commoner skin diseases treated?

Acne is a recurrent infection of the sebaceous glands, characterized by pustules, blackheads and scarring. So many adolescents develop acne that it can be regarded as a normal condition, although this is not much consolation for the sufferer. The treatment is frequent washing and vigorous flannelling to unblock sebaceous glands. If this fails, oral tetracycline 250 mg 6 hourly can be effective, as it kills the bacteria which proliferate in the blocked glands. Before prescribing tetracycline it is essential to ensure that the patient is not pregnant. The other measure which is effective in acne is ultraviolet light, either from the sun or via a sun lamp.

Psoriasis is a chronic scaling skin disease which is inherited, and affects 1 in 50 of the population. The lesions are red and scaly and are particularly found on extensor surfaces like the elbows. The disease comes and goes and the most effective treatment is the local application of cold tar ointment or salicylic acid ointment. Local steroids are effective, but their long-term use causes the skin to grow thin and delicate. Very bad psoriasis can be treated by cytotoxic drugs, since the scaling is due to overgrowth of the epidermis. A typical regime would be a single dose of methotrexate 10–30 mg every 14 days. Again this should not be given to pregnant women.

Eczema is an inflammatory disease with swelling, weeping and crusting of the skin, which becomes dry and cracked. Eczema is also familial, and associated with other allergic disorders such as asthma and hay fever. Patients have delicate skin which is worsened by anything which removes the oil from the skin. Soap should be avoided and oils and creams used as substitutes. Patches of eczema may respond to coal tar ointment or weak steroid creams.

What is the place of steroid creams in skin disease?

Steroid creams are very effective at reducing skin inflammation and itching. However, they are probably over-prescribed and patients with chronic skin diseases use them more than is advisable. Steroids have three main disadvantages:

(1) in infected skin they can cause spread of the infection,
(2) when used repeatedly steroids can cause skin atrophy,
(3) when used over a wide area sufficient steroid can be absorbed from the skin to cause suppression of the adrenal gland and other side-effects of systemic steroids.

What antibiotics can be used on skin?

Most skin infections are best treated with oral antibiotics. Penetration of the drug to the sites of infection is more reliable, and for some reason, local application of antibiotics very rapidly leads to sensitization and an allergic reaction. Penicillins should never be used topically. Chlortetracycline and gentamicin are available as local ointments for infected lesions. Clioquinol cream is also useful in infected lesions, such as impetigo.

What about anti-fungal agents?

Fungal infection of the skin, such as athlete's foot, ringworm and tinea cruris are common. Local application of an anti-fungal cream is usually effective, provided the patient does not become re-infected from their clothing. Whitfield's ointment is a traditional anti-fungal ointment which is a mixture of salicylic acid and benzoic acid. Zinc undecanoate is also effective and can be used as a powder. An important point, which is not often made, is that the patient should be warned not to apply such ointments to the sensitive skin of the genitals as this can be extremely painful. Persistent fungal infections, particularly those of the nails, have to be treated by systemic anti-fungal drugs such as griseofulvin 250 mg twice daily, and the course of treatment has to be prolonged because the nail grows very slowly.

What about the sterilization of skin?

Normal skin is covered with vast numbers of bacteria. Simple washing with soap and water diminishes their numbers considerably, but the skin is still not sterile. In aseptic technique the skin is washed in an iodine-containing disinfectant and then covered with a sterile adhesive film.

Traditionally, the skin is cleaned in an antiseptic solution before any injection is made or blood drawn; the usual choice here is an alcohol such as surgical spirit. It is best to remember that the skin should be allowed to dry after alcohol is used before being punctured. If a needle is passed into the skin via a pool of alcohol the needle prick is extremely painful. Similarly, after withdrawing a needle from the skin haemostasis should be secured not with an alcohol swab but with a clean cotton wool ball.

What is EUSOL?

EUSOL stands for Edinburgh University Solution of Lime and is a mixture of chlorinated lime and boric acid. EUSOL is a very useful agent, which is used to irrigate wounds and cavities and clean up festering ulcers.

How can itching be relieved?

Wetting the skin and cooling it by allowing a lotion to dry on it relieves itching. Calamine lotion is most frequently used. Oral antihistamines can also relieve itching at the cost of some sedation. In jaundice there may be intolerable itching, but this is due to bile salt deposition in the skin. An effective treatment is oral cholestyramine resin which binds bile salts in the gut, and increases their elimination. Cholestyramine is, however, rather unpleasant to take.

What side-effects can drugs cause in the skin?

Most commonly drugs cause a rash, and indeed drug rashes are the most common complication of drug therapy. Almost any type of skin eruption can be mimicked by drugs. Drug rashes are commonly of rapid onset, often vivid and extensive rather than localized. Some drugs very commonly cause rashes and for example ampicillin rash has a characteristic appearance which is readily recognizable. In any patient with a skin lesion drugs should be thought of as a possible cause.

Other common side-effects produced by drugs in the skin include acne, eczema, erythema nodosum (large painful lumps under the skin, particularly on the shins), pigmentation, purpura or bleeding.

29

Drugs and the eye

What are the commonest causes of blindness?

In the UK the commonest causes of blindness are chronic simple glaucoma, cataract, diabetic retinopathy and disciform senile macular degeneration. Of these relatively common diseases only diabetic retinopathy and chronic simple glaucoma have an effective drug treatment, and ophthalmology is a surgically orientated discipline.

How are diabetic retinopathy and simple glaucoma treated?

Diabetic retinopathy is treated in two ways. First, by meticulous attention to blood sugar control, and secondly, by photocoagulation of the abnormal retinal vessels which cause this condition. Simple glaucoma is treated with measures to reduce intraocular pressure, such as pupil constricting drugs and oral treatment with acetazolamide, a drug which reduces the rate of secretion of the aqueous humour.

How are drugs used in eye treatment?

Drugs are generally used by local installation into the eye, and rarely by systemic administration.

What drugs are used as eye drops?

Eye drops are used to dilate or constrict the pupil, as local anaesthetics, as antibiotics and as anti-inflammatory drugs. Dilatation of the pupil is used for examining it, and as treatment in inflammatory disease of the anterior eye such as uveitis. There are two different ways of dilating the pupil, either by stimulating the sympathetic system or blocking the cholinergic parasympathetic system. Neutral adrenaline or phenylephrine is used as an active sympathomimetic dilator of the pupil, and homatropine, atropine or tropicamide are used as passive anticholinergic dilators of the pupil. Tropicamide is the most rapidly acting of these, and is useful in eye clinics for examination of the retina.

Drugs which constrict the pupil are used in the treatment of glaucoma, the only exception being thrombotic glaucoma in diabetics. The usual drug employed is pilocarpine. When the pupil is constricted in this way intraocular pressure is reduced, and this is an effective way of managing glaucoma where vision is lost because of increased intraocular pressure.

Local anaesthetic drops on the cornea are used to aid examination of the eye. Amethocaine is the local anaesthetic commonly used.

What about the treatment of conjunctivitis?

Antibiotic drugs and antiviral drugs can be used to treat infections of the conjunctiva and cornea. The usual antibiotic employed is chloramphenicol. Chloramphenicol is an effective antibiotic, which is no longer used frequently as an oral drug, as it has an unacceptably high complication rate of aplastic anaemia. However, when given locally to the eye, little is absorbed and this is a very remote danger. Other antibiotics used include neomycin and sulphacetamide. Idoxuridine eye drops are a specific treatment for herpetic infections of the anterior eye.

When are steroid eye drops used?

Steroids are used to suppress inflammatory processes within the eye. They have a hazard in that they can lead to infections in the eye, but this is usually guarded against by giving them in combination with an antibiotic. They should *never* be used in patients who have a viral infection of the eye. Any steroid can be used but dexamethazone is one of the most powerful and effective.

When are systemic drugs used in the treatment of eye disease?

Systemic drugs are rather infrequently used in ophthalmology. Infections of the eye are not very effectively treated with systemic antibiotics as penetration into the eye is very slow. Systemic steroids are occasionally used in inflammatory conditions such as choroiditis and are very important in temporal arteritis. In this disease sudden blindness is a complication, and this can be prevented by prior diagnosis and maintenance treatment with steroids. Clofibrate, the anticholesterol drug, is occasionally used for treating exudates of cholesterol seen on the retina where these interfere with vision.

SECTION 9

WARD THERAPEUTICS

30

Drugs and emergencies

What drug administration can cause an emergency?

Emergencies can arise if a patient is allergic to a drug, particularly if he has received it by injection. Anaphylactic collapse resembles a faint with a precipitous fall in blood pressure, bronchoconstriction and sometimes laryngeal oedema. The collapse can occur immediately after an intravenous injection or within an hour of an intramuscular injection.

The treatment is critical. The patient should be laid down and given the following drugs:

(1) Intramuscular adrenaline, 1 ml of 1 in 1000 solution
(2) Intravenous antihistamine, e.g. chlorpheniramine 10 mg
(3) Intravenous hydrocortisone, 100 mg

What other emergencies can occur?

Most of the other emergencies consist of an exaggerated response to the drugs given, for example after vasodepressor or hypotensive drugs the blood pressure can fall precipitously, and this can produce a collapse or even a stroke. With a precipitous fall in blood pressure an important measure is to raise the patient's legs to increase venous filling of the heart. Another possible adverse effect from drug administration is loss of consciousness. This is particularly important where a patient has been put on mixtures of sedatives and analgesics, the depressant effects of which can be synergistic. Patients, particularly elderly ones, can lapse into coma if overtreated with sedative drugs.

Can errors in drug administration cause emergencies?

Giving a patient the wrong drug or the wrong dose of a drug can be disastrous, especially if the error is not noticed immediately, and particularly if the drug is given by injection. Some injections are particularly dangerous if given in error. For example:

(1) Potassium chloride injection. Ampoules of this solution are supplied for dilution in large volumes of intravenous fluid for administration. Fatal accidents have occurred when KCl has been mistaken for NaCl and used to dissolve intravenous injections. Death here is due to cardiac arrest.

(2) Digoxin injection. This preparation is now rarely used, as fatal accidents have occurred when the drug was administered in error having been substituted for another, particularly in children.

(3) Diamorphine. Any depressant drug, opiate, barbiturate, benzodiazepine, can be fatal in patients with respiratory failure. It sometimes happens that these patients are given a respiratory stimulant, doxapram, to stimulate breathing. In such circumstances, substitution of any depressant drug for this stimulant preparation can be fatal, and drugs such as diazepam and diamorphine do have similar names.

It is obvious from the above, and on general grounds, that any injection, particularly an intravenous injection, should always be checked by another person before administration.

What drugs should be kept for emergency use?

This obviously depends on the location. In specialized units dealing with viral disease or leukaemia, special emergencies arise. However, in a general ward common emergencies include cardiac arrest, epileptic fits, left ventricular failure and anaphylaxis. The minimum of injectable drugs for dealing with these emergencies should be kept available in the emergency tray. The selection should include atropine, isoprenaline and calcium gluconate for dealing with cardiac emergencies, diazepam injection for epileptic fits, aminophylline and frusemide injection for left ventricular failure and hydrocortisone, adrenaline and chlorpheniramine for anaphylaxis. This list of emergency drugs is likely to vary from place to place, but everyone working in a ward should know where the tray is and what is on it.

What is a cardiac arrest?

Cardiac arrest is a sudden failure of the circulation when the heart ceases to pump blood. The heart may just stop or beat in a disordered rhythm so that it ceases to be an effective pump. When this happens the patient loses consciousness, no pulse can be felt, regular breathing stops and the pupils become dilated. At this point the patient is now dead and will remain dead if the circulation cannot be maintained within a few minutes. If the brain is not resupplied with oxygenated blood after a period of 3 or 4 minutes then irreversible brain death occurs.

How is cardiac arrest treated?

This is a real emergency. First the circulation and respiration must be restarted and then measures must be taken to get the heart going again. Two measures are vital: compression of the heart and artificial ventilation. In practice the patient must be flung onto any hard surface, if necessary the floor, and forceful depression of the lower sternum begun using the overlapping palms of the hand and pushing with the operator's body weight. In this way the heart is compressed between the sternum and the backbone. However, circulating unoxygenated blood is clearly useless so the lungs must be inflated, and each artificial breath must be alternated with three or four cardiac compressions. The lungs are best ventilated by an intratracheal tube and an anaesthetic bag, but before the cardiac call team arrive to do this ventilation must be started either by mouth to mouth or preferably with an airway of the Brook type.

How is the heart restarted?

Occasionally the heart starts spontaneously following cardiac compression. Usually, however, some active treatment is necessary, and this must be preceded by an ECG trace to determine what rhythm the heart is in. If there is ventricular fibrillation then the treatment of choice is an electrical defibrillation from the shock trolley. If there is no electrical activity then the heart is in asystole and some intracardiac stimulant such as calcium chloride or adrenaline is necessary. An intravenous drip of sodium bicarbonate to correct acidosis is usually run in at this time. If some electrical activity can be restored, then more drugs can be given to convert the heart back to sinus rhythm.

What is the outcome of most cardiac arrests?

The outcome for most cardiac arrests in the general medical ward is poor. Most of the patients who have a cardiac arrest have obviously got some underlying abnormality which militates against their recovery. However, in younger patients with a more transient cardiac problem, particularly myocardial infarction, there is a better chance of good outcome.

What is an overdose?

In many centres, perhaps 10% of medical admissions are patients who have taken a deliberate overdose of drugs. Most of these patients are not trying to commit suicide, but are making a gesture of despair and indulging in a grim form of attention seeking. Despite the irritations one feels with dealing with these patients it must be remembered that all of them are ill and needing help.

How is a drug overdosage treated?

Contrary to popular opinion, few drugs have effective antidotes. The elimination of most drugs from the body cannot be accelerated by medical means. In short, nothing active can be done about most drug overdosage. The strategy in dealing with these patients is to use general measures to keep the patient alive until he eventually metabolizes and excretes the drug and recovers from its effects.

What general measures are used?

Most poisonings cause unconsciousness, depression of respiration and shock. When unconscious, the patient has to be cared for as in any case of coma, turned to prevent bed sores and nerve compression, exercised to prevent contractions and kept dry. Fluid intake has to be sufficient to maintain urinary output and electrolytes in good order. Depression of respiration may be severe enough to necessitate tracheal intubation and artificial ventilation. Shock, manifested by falling blood pressure, is more difficult to treat, and unless there is evidence that the circulation is failing so badly that tissue perfusion is inadequate, treatment is restricted to fluid replacement.

What about measures to increase elimination of the drug?

Once the drug has been absorbed there is little that can be done. Washing out the stomach with a tube or making the patient vomit is often practised. Such measures do little good, except in aspirin overdose where absorption of the drug is very slow and a proportion of the dose can be recovered if the stomach contents are vomited. In fact, stomach washouts are used in drug overdosage for two reasons, neither of which is legitimate. The first is to impress the coroner or relatives that something active is being done, and the second is to punish the patient for taking the drug.

Some drugs are eliminated from the body by the kidney rather than being metabolized by the liver. Such drugs can be eliminated more rapidly if the patient has a high urinary output. In severe cases of poisoning with certain drugs it is possible to enhance elimination of the drug by diuresis, and in other cases it is even possible to eliminate the drug by haemodialysis. However, these are rather desperate measures.

What about antidotes?

A few drugs do have specific antidotes. Iron poisoning can be actively treated with desferrioxamine a drug which chellates or takes up the metal ions. The effect of opiate overdosage can be antagonized with naloxone, a specific antagonist, which can induce opiate withdrawal in addicts.

One recent successful treatment has been the use of acetylcysteine in the treatment of paracetamol overdose. Acetylcysteine combines with the reactive metabolite of paracetamol which is responsible for the liver damage in patients poisoned with this drug.

Is it really important to find out what the patient has taken?

Knowledge of what the patient has taken is useful in predicting what is likely to happen to the patient, in deciding whether any specific treatment is available, or whether any means of eliminating the drug are worthwhile. Usually by far the most useful source of information is the patient and those he lives with. Faced with a completely unconscious, uncooperative patient, it is possible for chemical analysis to determine what the patient has taken, but this is a difficult matter and information is not usually available in time to make use of it.

31

Drugs and regulations

What legal regulations are there about the use of drugs?

In most countries the availability of drugs is regulated by law. The details differ but most countries recognize three main categories of drugs, those that can be sold directly to the public, those which are only supplied on the prescription of a doctor, and dangerous addictive drugs to which special regulations apply.

What laws govern drug usage in the UK?

Laws governing the use of drugs in the UK have changed in recent years. Certain old statutes such as the Pharmacy and Poisons Act of 1933 have been repealed and no longer apply. New regulations have been brought into force. The main acts which govern the supply of medicines are the Medicines Act of 1968, the Misuse of Drugs Act of 1971 and the Poisons Act of 1972.

How are drugs legally classified in the UK?

There are three classes of medicine:

(1) General Sales List (GSL). This list includes 'over-the-counter' medicines such as aspirin and cold cures, which can be sold directly to the public without record. Certain regulations as to labelling of these products, quantities available for sale and where they can be sold do apply.

(2) Pharmacy Medicines (P). Certain drugs can be sold to the public without prescription and without any record being made, but they have to be sold under the direction of a pharmacist. This places some restriction on their supply and gives the opportunity for the pharmacist to give advice to the patient who requests the drug.

(3) Prescription Only Medicines (POM). These drugs can only be supplied on prescription and records are kept of the drugs supplied and to whom. In an emergency, the pharmacist is empowered to supply a patient with up to 3 days supply of such a medicine, as for example when a patient runs out of a medicine which he takes regularly and it has been difficult for him to obtain another prescription. Certain POMs include controlled drugs to which further, more detailed, regulations apply.

What about dangerous drugs?

The Misuse of Drugs Act of 1971 replaces the Dangerous Drugs Regulations previously in force and establishes a new category of drugs, the controlled drug. These controlled drugs largely replace the old and more familiar 'DDAS'. The Act defines these drugs and lays down precise ways in which they must be stored and supplied. The drugs are so designated because they are liable to be misused. There are four different schedules of controlled drugs but the most important of these are schedules 2 and 4. Schedule 2 drugs are those such as the narcotic analgesics, amphetamines and other drugs which produce important dependence (Table 4). Schedule 4 drugs are not medical drugs but are those substances usually known as 'street drugs', including cannabis leaf, coca leaf, mescaline and the crude opiates.

Table 4 Controlled drugs listed in Schedule 2 of the Misuse of Drugs Act 1971. Certain formulations of these drugs are exempted, e.g. codeine and dihydrocodeine tablets, and morphine in the form of kaolin and morphine mixture

Amphetamine	Methaqualone
Chlorphentermine	Mephentermine
Cocaine	Methadone
Codeine	Methylamphetamine
Dexamphetamine	Methylphenidate
Dextromoramide	Morphine
Diamorphine	Nicocodine
Diethylthiambutene	Nicodicodine
Difenoxin	Opium
Dihydrocodeine	Oxycodone
Dihydrocodeinone	Papaveretum
Dipipanone	Pethidine
Drotebanol	Phenazocine
Fentanyl	Phenmetrazine
Hydrocodone	Phenoperidine
Hydromorphone	Piritramide
Levorphanol	Propiram

What do these controlled drugs regulations mean in practice?

In practice, controlled drugs must be stored and dispensed according to certain regulations. Such drugs must be kept in a locked cupboard and a record kept of their supply and use. Administration of a controlled drug to a patient has to be more elaborate than when any other POM is used, the main differences being:

(1) The prescription has to have the dose of the drug written in both words and figures, e.g. diamorphine five milligrams, 5 mg. The dose form, i.e. injection, linctus, etc., must be stated.

(2) The administration has to be recorded in the book kept for that purpose, i.e. the Controlled Drugs Book. Supplies of controlled drugs have to be ordered from the pharmacy by the wards in a separate book, and ward stocks of controlled drugs have to be checked by pharmacists at least every 3 months.

What about giving controlled drugs to an addict?

The Misuse of Drugs Act of 1971 requires addicts to be registered. Once an addict is so registered it is an offence for anyone to supply him with drugs for his addiction except via a special licensed treatment centre.

What about the administration of drugs on the ward?

The Medicines Act provides that no-one may administer a POM other than the patient himself, unless that person is under the direction of a medical practitioner. In practice this means that no drug must be administered without a valid prescription.

What constitutes a valid prescription?

A valid prescription must be written in ink, must be dated and signed. It must contain the name and address of the patient and the address of the doctor. However, in hospital these addresses need not be included on the valid prescription, but the patient's hospital case number must be on the sheet.

Can a laxative or an analgesic be given when it has not been prescribed?

All hospitals have their own local policy about these matters, but in general laxatives and analgesics of certain simple sorts are administered at the discretion of the ward staff.

How are medicines ordered for a ward?

Some hospitals operate a ward pharmacy system where a pharmacist visits a ward and arranges a supply of drugs. In other cases, orders have to be sent to the pharmacy by the ward, either in the form of an order book or the patient's individual treatment sheets which are sent down to the pharmacy. In the case of controlled drugs a special order book is used.

Must all medicines be locked away?

Yes this is good practice, the usual exceptions being topical lotions, drugs on the emergency trolley and medicines actually in use. Some drugs have to be stored in a refrigerator, and it is good practice to have a separate refrigerator for this purpose. Injections such as heparin and insulin have to be refrigerated.

Does the administration of all medicine have to be recorded?

No oral or injectable medicine should be given without a record being made. In most hospitals this is done on the patient's own prescription sheet, the nurse signing for each administration.

What happens if a patient refuses to take a medicine?

If a patient refuses to take a medicine then obviously this fact is recorded, and the nurse in charge and the doctor treating the patient are informed.

What should be done with the medicines which a patient may bring with him into the hospital?

Once dispensed by a retail pharmacist, the medicines are the property of the patient, but what is done in most hospitals is to lock the patient's medicines away on the ward together with the patient's valuables. The patient's permission must be obtained if they are sent back to the pharmacy if the treatment is being changed.

Can nurses give intravenous drugs?

Local policies on this differ, but in general intravenous injections can be given by nurses only into infusions or catheters which have already been placed in the vein. Most intravenous injections are given by medical staff. As regards the addition of drugs to bags of intravenous fluid, it is regarded as good policy if this is carried out actually in the pharmacy, where better sterile facilities are available for these additions.

What should be done if an error in dispensing drugs is made?

It is important that mistakes should be recorded, and that those looking after the patients should be informed. In all hospitals there is a procedure for reporting accidents to patients, and this should be followed in the case of a mistake in the administration of a drug.

Index

acne *see* skin diseases
addiction 81 *see also* dependence
administration, drug 10
  convenience 11
  effectiveness 11
  errors in 174
  hospital, in 172
  I.V., by nurses 173
  patient refusal 173
  recording 173
  route of 10
  safety of 12
  selectivity 11
  speed of action 11–12
adrenaline 92–93
  adrenal gland, release by 92, 117
  pharmacological actions 92–93
  receptors *see* adrenergic receptors
  sympathetic nervous system, in 92
adrenergic receptors,
  adrenaline, effect on 92–93
  alpha 92
  beta 92
  beta blocking drugs *see* beta blocking drugs
  drug action on 93
  noradrenaline, effect on 93
adverse drug effects 17–21
  allergy *see* allergy
  control of 21
  cumulative toxicity 19
  detection of 20–21
  exaggerated therapeutic effect 18
  idiosyncrasy 20
  importance of 17
  side effects 18–19
  toxic effect 19
  types of 17–18
  WHO definition 17
  see also named drugs
allergy 19–20, 38–39
  anaphylaxis *see* anaphylaxis
  antibiotic induced *see* antibiotics
  desensitization 39
  immune system, and 38–39
  mechanism 19–20, 38
  prevention 38–39
  X ray contrast media induced 20
amoebiasis *see* tropical diseases
anaemia 147–149
  daily iron requirement 147
  dietary iron intake 147
  haematinics 147–149
    folic acid 148
    iron 148
    vitamin B_{12} 148, 149
  iron deficiency 147–148
    causes 147
    effects of 148
    incidence 147
    treatment 148
  oral iron 148
    dosage 148
    side effects 148
anaesthetics 54–59
  administration 58
  gaseous 57–58
    hazards of 58
    mode of action 57–58
  general 54
  induction by 54, 55
  muscle relaxants *see* muscle relaxants
  patient preparation for 54–55
  premedication 54, 55
  stages of anaesthesia 59
analgesics 60–64
  administration without prescription 172
  definition 60
  endorphins and 62

narcotic 60–63
addiction 61–62
antagonists 63
mode of action 62
morphine *see* morphine
types 60–61, 62
usage 60
minor 63
arthritis, in 64
aspirin 63
mode of action 63
paracetamol 63
prostaglandins and *see* prostaglandins
side effects 64
anaphylaxis,
drug induced 19, 20
immune system and 38
treatment 165
vaccine induced 40
antibiotics 27–33
bacterial resistance to 29
broad spectrum 28
cephalosporins 32
classification 27–28
contraceptive pill and 31
co-trimoxazole 33
penicillin *see* penicillins
prophylactic 29–30
selection 28
side effects 30–31
sulphonamides 33
tetracyclines 32
anticoagulants 150–153
antiplatelet agents 152–153
contraindications 152
definition 150
drug interactions 152
heparin 150–151
indications 151
oral 150–151
anticonvulsants 68–70
carbamazepine 70
epilepsy *see* epilepsy
indications 69
mode of action 68–69
phenobarbitone 70
phenytoin 69–70
principles of therapy 69
sodium valproate 70
antihypertensives 95–101
adrenergic neurone blockers 99
beta blockers 99, 99–100
centrally acting 100–101
diuretics 99, 100
ganglion blockers 99
mild hypertension, in 99
severe hypertension, in 100
vasodilators 99
see also hypertension
anxiety *see* psychotropic drugs
aspirin *see* analgesics
asthma 108–110
bronchodilators 108–109
atropine-like drugs 109
beta mimetic drugs 108–109
theophylline 109
cromoglycate 109
definition 108
mucolytics 110
prognosis 110
status asthmaticus 110
steroids 109
treatment 108
autonomic nervous system 87–110
definition 87
importance 87–88
parasympathetic 88–91
drug effects on 90–91
neurotransmitters 90
structure 88–89
sympathetic 88–89, 92
neurotransmitters 92
receptors *see* adrenergic receptors

barbiturates,
epilepsy, in 69–70
hypnotics, as 66, 67
side effects 66–67
benzodiazepines
anxiety, in 73–74
hypnotics, as 66, 67
beta blocking drugs 93–94
side effects 94
usage 93–94
see also cardiac disease, hypertension
blood *see* anaemia, anticoagulants
brain 51–53
drug action on 52
function 51
neurotransmitters *see* neurotransmitters

cancer 44
chemotherapy *see* cancer chemotherapy
definition 44

cancer chemotherapy 44–48
alkylating agents 45
antimetabolites 45
cell division and 48
chromosome inhibitors 45
drug regimes 46–47
efficacy 46
hormones 47
local infusions 47
principle 44–45
radioactive drugs 45–46
side effects 46, 47
cardiac disease 102–107
acute myocardial infarction 107
angina 106–107
beta blockers 107
calcium antagonists 107
definition 106
nitrites 106
cardiac arrhythmias 104–106
beta blockers 106
classification 105
definition 104–105
local anaesthetics 105–106
quinidine-like drugs 106
coronary heart disease 106–107
heart failure 102–104
catecholamine-like drugs 102–103
definition 102
digitalis glycosides *see* digitalis glycosides
central nervous system 51–84
brain *see* brain
drugs and 52
neurotransmitters *see* neurotransmitters
chemotherapy 25–48
cancer *see* cancer chemotherapy
definition 27
immune system and *see* immune system
infectious diseases, of *see* infectious diseases
mode of action 27
tropical diseases, of *see* tropical diseases
tuberculosis, of *see* tuberculosis
cholera *see* tropical diseases
cigarettes *see* tobacco smoking
conjunctivitis *see* eye diseases

dependence, drug,
alcohol 82
caffeine 82, 84
definition 81
hypnotics 65, 66–67
narcotics 61
nicotine 82
depression 74–76
antidepressants 75–76
monoamine oxidase inhibitors 75–76
tricyclics 75
endogenous 74
manic 74
reactive 74
suicide and 74
diabetes mellitus 119–123
blood glucose and 120
causes 120
clinical types 119
definition 119
diabetic coma in 122
diet, role of 120
eye checking in 123
insulin 120, 121–122
mechanism 119
oral hypoglycaemics 122
sulphonylureas 122
treatment 120
digestive system, drugs and 139–144
antacids 141
anti-nauseants 143
constipation 143–144
duodenal ulcer 139–141
causes 139
incidence 139
treatment 140, 142
dyspepsia 139
gallstones 142
gastric bleeding, drug induced 142
gastric reflux 141
gastric ulcer 141, 142
purgatives 144
digitalis glycosides 103–104
digitalis 103
digitoxin 104
oubain 104
strophanthin 104
diuretics 135–138
classification 135
definition 135
indications 135
loop 137
mechanism of action 135–136
potassium sparing 137–138
thiazide 136–137

dosage, drug 7–9
  interindividual variation 8–9
  interval 7–8
  plasma concentrations, and 7–8, 9
  therapeutic range 9
drug,
  absorption 6
  administration *see* administration, drug
  classification 16, 170–171
  definition 3
  development 12–13
  dosage *see* dosage, drug
  distribution 6
  elimination 6
  formulation 12
  half life 8
  interaction 10–11
  mode of action 3–6
  names 14–16
  receptors *see* receptor
  regulations *see* drug regulations
  transport 5
drug regulations 170–174
  controlled drugs 171–172
  dangerous drugs 171
  legal classification 170–171
  ordering drugs, and 173
  storing drugs, and 173
  U.K. laws 170
  valid prescription 172

eczema *see* skin diseases
emergencies 165–169
  cardiac arrest 166–167
    outcome 167
    symptoms 166
    treatment 167
  drug induced 165
    anaphylactic collapse *see* anaphylaxis
    exaggerated response 165
  drugs for 166
  error in drug administration 165–166
  overdose 167–169
    antidotes 168–169
    definition 167
    incidence 167
    increased drug elimination in 168
endocrine system 113–118
  adrenal gland 117
  classification 113–114
  drug treatment, effect of 113
  function 113
  parathyroid gland 118
  pituitary *see* pituitary hormones
  thyroid gland 116–117
epilepsy,
  definition 68
  drugs for *see* anticonvulsants
  refractory 70
  status epilepticus 70–71
eye diseases 161–162
  blindness, causes of 161
  conjunctivitis 162
  diabetic retinopathy 161
  eyedrops 161, 162
  systemic drugs 162

hypertension 95–101
  blood pressure, regulation of 97
  classification 95–96
  consequences of 95
  definition 95
  life expectancy and 96
  malignant 95–96, 101
  postural 99
  treatment 97 *see also* antihypertensives
hypnotics 65–67
  barbiturates 66–67
  benzodiazepines 66, 67
  definition 65
  dependence on 65, 66
  insomnia 65
  side effects 65–66
  types 65

immune system 38–43
  allergy, role in *see* allergy
  anti D antibody, and *see* rhesus disease
  passive immunity 38, 40–42
  stimulation of 38
    vaccines *see* vaccines
  suppression of 38
    immunosuppressants *see* immunosuppression
immunosuppression 42–43
  drugs for 42
    side effects 42–43
  principle 42
  renal transplantation, in 43
infectious diseases 25–33
  antibiotics in *see* antibiotics
  drugs for 26–27
  causative organisms 25–27
  prevention of 26
  treatment 26–27

see also named diseases, tropical diseases
insomnia *see* hypnotics

kidney,
diuretics *see* diuretics
drug elimination by 6
renal tubule anatomy 136

L-dopa, in Parkinson's disease 79–80
decarboxylase inhibitors 79–80
dose regime 79
efficacy 79
failure of response 80
principle 79
side effects 79
leprosy *see* tropical diseases

malaria *see* tropical diseases
mental disease *see* psychotropic drugs
Misuse of Drugs Act 171
morphine 60, 61–63
actions 61
antagonist 63
side effects 61
muscle relaxants 55–57
anaesthesia, in 55–56
curare-like drugs 56
depolarising 56–57
mode of action 56

nervous system 87
autonomic *see* autonomic nervous system
central *see* central nervous system
peripheral 87
neurotransmitters,
central 52–53
acetylcholine 53
amino acids 53
dopamine 52
noradrenaline 52
serotonin 53
imbalance in Parkinson's disease 78
parasympathetic 90
acetylcholine 90
sympathetic 92
adrenaline *see* adrenaline
acetylcholine 92
noradrenaline *see* noradrenaline
noradrenaline 92, 93
pharmacology 93
receptors *see* adrenergic receptors
sympathetic nervous system, in 92

oral contraception 124–127
contraindications 126
drug interactions 126
efficacy 124
mini-pill 126
oestrogen dose 126
principle 124–125
progestagen dose 126
side effects 125
triphasic pill 127
overdose *see* emergencies

Parkinson's disease 77–80
anticholinergic drugs in 78
cause 77
description 77
dopaminergic drugs in *see* L-dopa
drug induced 80
treatment 77–78
penicillins 31–32
allergy to 32
historical development 31
safety of 32
spectrum of activity 31–32
varieties of 31–32
pharmacodynamics 5
pharmacokinetics 6
pituitary hormones 114–116
anterior 114–116
adrenocorticotrophin(ACTH) 114
gonadotrophins 115
growth hormone(GH) 115
prolactin 115–116
thyrotropin(TSH) 115
posterior 114, 116
antidiuretic(ADH) 116
oxytocin 116
pregnancy, drugs in 128–132
early pregnancy 131–132
labour, in 131
morning sickness 132
post natal 132
prescribed drugs 132
teratogenesis *see* teratogenesis
prostaglandins 63
central nervous, in the 53
inflammation, and 63
inhibition of 63, 152
platelet aggregation, and 152–153
prostacyclin 153
psoriasis *see* skin diseases
psychotropic drugs 72–76
antipsychotics 72–73

anxiety, in 73–74
depression 75–76
mental disease, in 72
neurosis 72
psychosis 72

receptors 4–5
adrenergic *see* adrenergic receptors
drug-receptor interaction 4–5
drug structure, and 5
site of 5
rhesus disease 41
anti D antibody, and 41

schistosomiasis *see* tropical diseases
sedatives *see* hypnotics
skin diseases 157–160
acne 157–158
adverse drug effects 160
antibiotics in 158
antifungal agents in 159
drug application 157
eczema 158
EUSOL in 159
psoriasis 158
relief of itching 158–159
skin sterilization 159
steroid creams 158
smoking *see* tobacco smoking
social drugs 81–84
abuse 81
addiction *see* addiction
acceptance in society 81
coffee 82, 84
dependence *see* dependence
tea 82, 84
tobacco *see* tobacco smoking

teratogenesis 128–131
definition 128
drug induced 129–130
incidence 128
mechanism 130
prevention 130–131
selective toxicity 130
tobacco smoking 82–84
disease incidence and 82
life expectancy 82
low tar cigarettes 83–84
nicotine 82, 83, 84
absorption 82, 83
blood concentration 82
dependence 82
withdrawal phase 82
pharmacological basis of 82–83
psychological factors 82, 83
reducing cigarette consumption 83
topical therapy 157–162
definition 157
eye, of *see* eye diseases
skin, of *see* skin diseases
toxic effects *see* adverse drug effects
tropical diseases 36–37
amoebiasis 36
cholera 36–37
definition 36
leprosy 37
malaria 36
schistosomiasis 37
tuberculosis 34–36
chronicity 34
definition 34
forms 34
mortality 34
treatment 35–36

ulcers *see* digestive system, drugs and

vaccines 38–41
animal sera 41
anti D antibody *see* rhesus disease
contraindications 40
definition 39
hazards of 40
human antibodies 41
mode of action 39
passive immunity, and 38–41
routine 40
rubella 40

GPSR Compliance

The European Union's (EU) General Product Safety Regulation (GPSR) is a set of rules that requires consumer products to be safe and our obligations to ensure this.

If you have any concerns about our products, you can contact us on ProductSafety@springernature.com

In case Publisher is established outside the EU, the EU authorized representative is:

Springer Nature Customer Service Center GmbH
Europaplatz 3
69115 Heidelberg, Germany

Batch number: 10620169

Printed by Printforce, the Netherlands